100 *MORE* DAYS *of*

WEIGHT
LOSS

100 *MORE* DAYS *of*
WEIGHT
LOSS

Giving You the Power
to Be Successful on
Any Diet Plan

A DAILY MOTIVATOR

LINDA SPANGLE, RN, MA

SunQuest
Media

Published in Denver, Colorado, by SunQuest Media.
SunQuest Media titles may be purchased in bulk for educational, business
or sales promotional use. For ordering information, please visit
www.WeightLossJoy.com.

Manufactured in the United States of America
ISBN# 978-0-9767057-4-1
eBook ISBN# 978-0-9767057-5-8

10 9 8 7 6 5 4 3

Names: Spangle, Linda.
Title: 100 more days of weight loss : giving you the power to be successful
on any diet plan : a daily motivator / Linda Spangle, RN, MA.
Other Titles: One hundred more days of weight loss
Description: Denver, Colorado : SunQuest Media, [2018] | "Portions
of this book were excerpted from Life is Hard, Food is Easy by Linda
Spangle, and Linda's online newsletter, The Weight Loss Minute." |
Includes index.
Identifiers: ISBN 9780976705741 | ISBN 9780976705758 (ebook)
Subjects: LCSH: Reducing diets--Psychological aspects. | Weight loss--
Psychological aspects. | Motivation (Psychology) | Affirmations.
Classification: LCC RM222.2 .S675 2018 (print) | LCC RM222.2 (ebook) |
DDC 613.25--dc23

Cover photo by Michael Jung

The information in this book is not a substitute for medical or psychological
counseling and care. All matters pertaining to your physical or mental
health should be supervised by a physician or health-care professional.

Portions of this book were excerpted from *Life Is Hard, Food Is Easy* by
Linda Spangle, and Linda's online newsletter, *The Weight-Loss Minute*.

❧ CONTENTS ❧

DAYS 31-40 SUSTAIN MOTIVATION

DAYS 41-50 SEPARATE EMOTIONS AND FOOD

DAYS 51-60 FIX THE REAL NEEDS

DAYS 61-70 MANAGE EMOTIONS WITHOUT FOOD

DAYS 71-80 OVERCOME BARRIERS AND SABOTAGE

❧ WELCOME ❧

When Allison arrived at my office for her weekly meeting, she immediately pulled out her journal and a worn copy of the book *100 Days of Weight Loss*. "This is so amazing!" she said. "I can't even remember when I've stayed on a diet longer than a few weeks. But look at me! This time, I've lost 30 pounds, and it's partly because I've been solid on my program for almost three months!

"Now I'm ready to start the lessons in the new book *100 MORE Days of Weight Loss*. I know they'll keep me on track and help me maintain my weight-loss goals."

Allison's story is not unique. Using my daily motivational lessons has improved weight-loss progress for thousands of readers. Now it's time to deepen your skills for achieving long-term success.

100 MORE Days of Weight Loss will give you phenomenal learning and personal growth. But you'll also discover ways to overcome barriers such as emotional eating that get in the way of success. Most of all, this book will prepare you for maintaining your weight long-term.

It doesn't matter if you've read the first book in the series. The lessons in the *100 MORE Days* book will all apply to your current efforts. Of course, reading or reviewing the first *100 Days* book might be helpful as well.

Choose your plan

Because this book is designed to work with any diet plan, you get to choose your own method for losing weight. Pick your best program, group or weight-loss app, then use this book to help you stick with it for a minimum of 100 days. If you need help with choosing a diet plan, take the quiz at www.thedietquiz.com.

Plan to complete one lesson from this book each day, setting a goal of staying on your chosen weight-loss plan for 100 consecutive days. If that's not realistic or practical, you can space the lessons any way you want.

Track your progress

With each day's lesson, record your answers to the "Today" assignment as well as any other insights or ideas that will help you in the future. Use a special notebook or journal or choose an online method for tracking your program.

I suggest you also come up with a visual way to track your 100 days. You might write each day's number on a calendar or in your daily planner. For more ideas, be sure to sign up for the free materials for this book that include a printable journal and the popular Dot Calendar.

Seven keys to staying motivated

Weight-loss motivation is tricky. Often it's there one day and gone the next. But the most important thing is not whether you feel motivated every single day. Instead, it's your ability to revive motivation over and over when it slips away.

Here are seven keys to successfully completing the 100 lessons in this book as well as managing your weight long-term.

Go to www.100MoreDays.com to print the Seven Keys worksheet and fill in your answers for each of the steps. By the time you finish, you'll be totally fired up and ready to start 100 More Days.

Key #1 – Always move forward!

Your past does not determine your future. So it doesn't matter if you've fallen off your diet or gained weight back in the past. This is now!

Tell yourself that starting today, you are moving forward and never going back. Pump your fist in the air and proclaim, "From this moment on, I'm moving forward!" Then celebrate the beginning of your new life.

Key #2 – Do what worked before

Think about times when you have been successful in the past. What did you do? Was there a specific diet plan that worked? Did you get up early and exercise before going to work? Maybe you cooked more meals at home instead of eating at restaurants.

Make a list of specific things that worked for you before. Put a star or check mark beside the ones you plan to use during your 100 MORE days.

Key #3 – No more excuses

Think about all the reasons you haven't been making progress. Whine a bunch about why you can't lose weight or exercise regularly. Write down your biggest reasons, then read your list of excuses out loud

Listen to how weak they sound. Now tell yourself that none of them work any more. From now on, catch your excuses as soon as they come out of your mouth. Remind yourself they don't matter and you have to do your program anyway. Then go do it.

Key #4 – Create a finish line

Build a vision of how this project will look when you reach the end of this book. How will you look, feel, and act when you cross the 100 MORE Days finish line? In addition to your new weight, picture yourself having confidence, energy and renewed zest for life.

Create a visual image of the finish line for your weight loss efforts. Perhaps you could make a collage of your new life. Or pull out a favorite thin outfit or pair of jeans and hang it where you can see it often. Try it on every week or two and see how the fit is changing. Use it to remind yourself of where you plan to be in the days ahead.

Key #5 – Kick the roadblocks

Think about what gets in your way when you're working on losing weight. What might keep you from success? Is it related to people, energy, money? When you've struggled with this in the past, what caused you to slip up or kept you from making progress? Identify everything you can think of. Write them all down.

If you're brave, make a copy of the page, then crumple the paper into a ball and kick it around the room for a few minutes. Picture every one of the roadblocks as being gone. You can also type your list on the computer and then delete the roadblocks one at time. Cheer each time one goes away.

Key #6 – Line up a support system

It really helps if you have someone who cares about you and your efforts to complete the 100 MORE Days book. Get a buddy, hire a cheerleader or enlist your family members.

Key #7 – Learn and grow forever

The lessons in this book are only the beginning. For the months ahead, plan all the ways you can continue with your personal growth. Maybe you could read more books, take yoga or Pilates classes or hire a life coach or a personal trainer.

Never give up

At the end of each set of ten lessons, you'll find two divider pages that include a list of the next group of topics. If you ever feel tempted to stop your program, skip to one of these pages where you'll see the following message:

> ### You've come this far in your 100 days...
>
> *Don't stop now.* If you're struggling to stick with it, push yourself to finish one more day. You'll immediately be another day closer to achieving your weight-loss goals.
>
> ### Just do one more day!

Each time you complete another day on your 100 MORE Days Program, you'll have moved further on the road toward your new life. Stay dedicated to your dream—and make it a great 100 days!

❧ FREE MATERIALS ❧

Be sure to sign up for the free
support materials for this book.

www.100MOREdays.com

- 100 More Days printable journal
- 7 keys to successful weight loss
- Printable signs for lesson reminders
- Dot calendar for visually tracking your progress
- Extensive word list to help identify emotions

A printed version of

100 MORE Days of Weight Loss
Day-by-Day Journal

is available on www.amazon.com

❧ DAYS 1–10 ❧

SEE YOUR POTENTIAL

✎ DAY 1 ✎
Others have done it

I still remember the day Janet sank into my office chair and started to cry. "I'm so discouraged!" she said. "I've been trying forever to lose weight, but I'm not making any progress at all. In fact, lately I've been gaining again. Right now, reaching my goal weight feels impossible. I don't think it can be done and I'm ready to give up."

I'm sure you've felt this way at times, and like Janet, you've decided that losing weight or maintaining long-term is impossible. Maybe you never stick to your weight-loss plan or you lose motivation or you hate exercise. Perhaps you've dieted many times but you always gain the weight back. At some point, you conclude it can't be done!

Wait! It *can* be done! In spite of what you hear in the news or from your friends, weight-loss success happens all the time.

Starting today, cultivate a belief that you *can* be successful with managing your weight. Remind yourself that many other people have accomplished this, and so can you. Reinforce your belief by telling yourself this powerful message:

Others have done it and so can I!

Success stories are everywhere. Somehow, these people have figured it out. And trust me, it wasn't because they discovered some huge secret known to only a select few. Instead, they kept working at it, learning, focusing and moving forward with their goals—not just for a few days or weeks, but for months and even years.

Be inspired by others

Think about all the people you know. I'll bet you can identify at least one person who has been successful at losing weight and then maintaining a healthy weight long-term. If you can't recall any friends or family members who've done this, have a chat with a weight-loss coach or program leader. Or search for "weight-loss success stories" online.

You'll soon discover that thousands of people have done it. Instead of telling yourself it can't be done, draw inspiration from the success stories of the world. Model after what they've accomplished and remind yourself that *others have done it and so can I.*

TODAY

- Find several people who have been successful with losing or maintaining their weight. Ask them what they did and how they made it work.

- From their comments, write a list of three things you can apply to your own efforts.

- Make a sign that says, "Others have done it and so can I." Place it where you can read it often and let it inspire you to reach your goals.

꧁ DAY 2 ꧂

I'll start tomorrow

Day after day, Amy would mess up just a little on her weight-loss plan. Maybe she'd grab a couple of cookies from the break room or she'd feel too tired to exercise. Then she'd tell herself, "I'll start tomorrow when I can do it perfectly." Unfortunately, she never made much progress with losing weight.

Does this sound familiar? Or maybe you don't even reach that point. You keep intending to start a diet or set up an exercise plan, but it doesn't happen. First there were the holidays, the bad weather and spring break. Then you felt too tired to think about cooking and planning. But soon, you realize another season has slipped by, and your weight is the same as a year ago.

Of course, you're determined to work on your weight *some day*, but that day never comes. You keep postponing it for tomorrow or after the weekend or once school starts. Maybe you say, "After this is over, I'll get back on track." But then something else happens and stalls you again.

Maybe you convince yourself you can't lose weight right now because of the kids, an insensitive husband or boss, your back problem, even the weather. Or you tell yourself that nothing works anyway, so why bother?

Perhaps you minimize the problem. "It's not really so bad. There are other people worse off than I am. Besides, my weight isn't bothering me that much. My health is good for an overweight person."

Start NOW, not tomorrow

You can waste a lot of time and energy with "one of these days" intentions. So unless you're ready to take action, don't even utter the words. Be honest with yourself. If you aren't totally ready to lose weight right now, drop the guilt trip and wait until the time is right.

If you are determined to lose weight, then tackle it head-on. Get clear about your diet and exercise plans, then figure out how make them happen. Count your calories or your carbs. Ride your bike, take long walks, or go to the gym and do your workouts.

Don't wait for a day when you can be perfect. You need the benefits of losing weight NOW, not in a year or two. So follow through on your intentions and start *today*.

TODAY

- Identify one thing that is getting in the way of your weight-loss plan.

- Decide how you can get past this barrier. Write down your ideas.

- Take the steps that will make it happen today. Record what you did.

∾ DAY 3 ∾
What if I fail?

Trudy was scared! As we reviewed her new diet and exercise plan, she kept interrupting our discussion to remind me of her fears. "I hope I can make this work," she said. "I want to lose weight so badly this time. But I'm so worried. What if I can't do it?"

"What are you afraid of?" I asked. Her response was instant. "I'm afraid I'll fail again. I always start out strong, but then I get discouraged and quit. I'm scared I'll follow the same pattern."

Failure is such a negative word! Even if you have times when you struggle or gain some weight back, don't allow that awful word into your day. You have power over what happens in your life. So today, start conquering your fears by changing the way you think about them.

Emotions and logic

Your brain has an *emotional* side and a *logical* side. The emotional side panics a lot and pushes fear to the top of your thoughts. When you go through a hard time and totally mess up your plan, your emotional side celebrates. It knows you are about to give in and believe what it's telling you. Then it convinces you that, based on past experiences, your current plan will never work and, once again, you'll be a failure.

The logic side of your brain takes a totally different approach. It clarifies the facts, gives you insight and offers suggestions on how to take action against your fears. It also helps you learn from the past so you don't repeat your old patterns.

Push toward logic

Suppose you have eaten a big piece of chocolate cake or finished off a carton of ice cream. Which of these responses would be your first thought?

Emotional side: I've messed up big-time today. It's just like I thought. I'll never be successful with managing my weight.

Logical side: I had a difficult day, including some unplanned eating. I'm going to analyze what happened and make plans to prevent doing the same thing tomorrow.

With practice, you can learn how to catch it quickly when the emotional side is taking over. Do a fast analysis of what happened, then listen to your logic side and let go of your fears.

TODAY

- Write down one of your biggest fears around managing your weight.

- Identify your emotional response to it. Let yourself feel the fear and panic around it.

- Create a logical, positive message to use any time fears creep into your thoughts.

❧ DAY 4 ❧
Today I am on my plan

Imagine you are a parent and you have brought your toddler along when you went to the mall. Even while you are looking for the perfect outfit, you would still keep a close eye on your child. You certainly wouldn't get so preoccupied that you would forget you'd brought your child along.

Successful weight management requires a similar level of focus. As you go through your day, you need to always hold a subtle awareness of your plan and your healthy actions. And when you let up on your focus, especially during times you feel weak or vulnerable, it's a setup for disaster.

How we lose focus

Some years ago, I was invited to one holiday dinner with my family and another one a couple days later with a group of friends. During the meal with family members, I carefully monitored what I was eating. I savored and appreciated the tasty food but left a fair amount on my plate.

But at the second gathering, I somehow *forgot* to pay attention to my food intake. By the time the plates were cleared, I'd eaten way more than I'd intended. I pushed back from the table feeling stuffed, and a bit disgusted with myself for eating so much.

What went wrong? I didn't set out to overeat or ignore my diet. I simply lost my focus and stopped being aware of my eating plan.

Focus doesn't mean you can't have fun. Instead, it provides a way to remember your plan in spite of what's going

8

on around you. It's what keeps you from *forgetting* that you are striving to eat smaller portions, limit sweets or follow a specific food plan.

Keep focus strong

Start each day by saying, "Today, I am on my plan and I will stay on it all day!" Remind yourself often that you are determined to stay on your program. If you start slipping into old patterns, review your weight-loss goals and why they are important to you. Then intentionally renew your focus and push forward again.

Like any good parent, don't forget about your weight-loss efforts. Instead, develop a self-care antenna that helps you stay focused on how you want to live every single day.

TODAY

- Write a list of three things you will do to stay on your plan today.

- Identify any emotional issues such as stress that might get in the way of your focus.

- Create a self-talk phrase to use instantly when your focus starts to slip away.

❧ DAY 5 ❧
No willpower

As Dana settled into my office chair, I could sense her anger and frustration. "I had an awful weekend!" she began. "It started Friday when someone brought doughnuts to our weekly staff meeting. I ate one doughnut, then told myself that was it. But I couldn't resist them and pretty soon I grabbed another one."

"Wait a minute," I responded. "Two doughnuts ruined your whole weekend?"

Dana sighed. "No, if I'd stopped there, it wouldn't have been so bad. But after the meeting, I kept slipping into the break room until I'd eaten four more. After work, I went to my mom's and ate two pieces of chocolate layer cake." At this point, Dana looked up and said, "I know exactly what my problem is. I have no *willpower!*"

It's not my fault

What a great excuse! Lack of willpower means it's not your fault when you give in to the doughnuts or Mom's cake. While there are situations where willpower is important, it's never going to fix your weight-loss struggles.

The concept of willpower stems from a flawed belief that if you have this gift, you can resist any temptation. But in reality, willpower is not something you either *have* or *don't have*. Instead of worrying you won't be able to resist food temptations because of your weak willpower, create an instant plan or *mindset* for managing them.

A new mindset

Before you enter the room for a meeting, mentally rehearse how you'll manage the situation. Ask yourself, "What can I do to protect myself from the tempting food?" Then eat a healthy snack right before the meeting, sit at the end of the table farthest from the doughnut box, and sip on a cup of herbal tea. You'll quickly see that willpower isn't necessary when you use a mindset of protecting yourself.

Anytime you suddenly face a challenging event, reach for the tools that you know have worked in the past. Go brush your teeth, leave the room, postpone eating. Do anything that will help you stay strong and focused on your goals.

If you believe you can manage your actions by the choices you make, you won't have to worry about willpower abandoning you at the wrong moment. Instead, just pull another item from your strategy list and face down the food temptation without a hitch.

TODAY

- Think about places where you'll face a food temptation today.

- Create a new mindset for protecting yourself from unplanned eating.

- Record your success with using this new mindset.

ᔋ DAY 6 ᔍ
Monday diet

As the weekend approaches, you tell yourself, "This time I'm sticking with my diet and not messing it up." But by Friday afternoon, life has taken a toll.

Maybe you're physically exhausted or emotionally worn down from the week. Perhaps your daily battles with stress, depression or loneliness have caught up with you. So you seek a bit of solace, and food does the job perfectly.

By bedtime on Friday, you've eaten three days' worth of carbs or calories, but then who's counting anyway! At this point, you figure you've blown your diet and might as well enjoy the weekend. You can always start over on Monday.

What goes wrong?

I don't think this Monday-morning syndrome is caused by the wrong diet or not having enough motivation. I think it's related to the human condition and the way we seek pleasure, nurturing and comfort.

By the weekend, your emotional bucket is usually drained pretty low. And unless you stop for a refill, you'll easily slip into reaching for food as an easy fix. Before long, you routinely follow the pattern of *weekend pig-out, Monday diet.*

Fill your heart back up

Instead of trying to make your diet plan more rigid or isolating yourself from social events, consider ways you can take care of your heart.

Before next Friday, look at your schedule for the weekend. Make note of any social events, your children's sports or lessons, and family time. Identify the high-risk places where you tend to cross the line and give up on your diet plan.

Decide how you'll stick with your food and exercise goals as well as get some emotional refueling. Then build these ideas into a written plan that starts on Friday afternoon and ends on Sunday evening. Tape this to your refrigerator or the dashboard in your car.

Next weekend, don't go off your diet because you're emotionally empty. Instead, take care of your heart by doing the activities on your plan. If you do this every weekend, you won't need to regroup and start your diet over again on Monday.

TODAY

- Look at your schedule for next weekend and note any social events, as well as places where you tend to need rest, comfort or nurturing.

- Create a weekend revival plan. Write it down and tape it to your refrigerator, your computer or the dashboard in your car.

- Beginning on Friday afternoon, follow your special plan and take care of your heart's needs. Record how things went.

∾ DAY 7 ∾
Not willing to change

Cheryl was discouraged because this was the third week she hadn't lost any weight. As we reviewed her food journal, I was puzzled about why she wasn't losing. From Sunday to Thursday, her calorie level was within her goal range and she'd exercised almost every day.

"What's this note about Friday evening?" I asked. "All it says is FORGET IT!"

Cheryl looked a bit sheepish. "Every Friday after work, I meet a group of friends at this great neighborhood restaurant. I plan to be careful about what I eat, but after a couple of drinks, I go along with everyone else and have a good time. I know my calorie intake is probably out of sight, so I don't even write it down."

"Interesting," I said. "So your Friday night party sort of cancels out your efforts of the rest of the week." Cheryl groaned and said, "I know. But I've met with this group almost every Friday night for a couple of years. I guess I'm just not willing to give it up."

What are you *not* willing to do?

Unfortunately, Cheryl's need to join the party every Friday created a major roadblock in her weight-loss plan. Of course, she's not alone.

In your eating and exercise goals, what are you *not* willing to do? What do you keep holding on to, even though it affects your weight loss or ability to maintain? Are there certain foods or activities you just can't give up? Or maybe some things seem too hard, so you drag your feet on making important changes in your life.

Shift just a little

You don't have to eliminate all of these areas at once. Instead, identify one issue at a time and look for ways to compromise just a little. A tiny bit of extra effort is often enough to change your pattern. For example, if you're not willing to exercise, maybe you could walk for five minutes or go to the end of your street and back.

In Cheryl's plan, she decided to join her friends an hour later as a way to skip her usual margaritas and appetizers. That small change cut out a lot of calories as well as helped her make better choices on her meal. She also loved not having to start over again every Monday.

TODAY

- Identify several things you are not willing to do.

- Decide how you could make small changes in those areas and get past them.

- Record your new plan and follow through with it today.

ᔐ DAY 8 ᔑ

Set *now* goals

Sara wanted to lose 100 pounds but she always felt over-whelmed with the prospect. Since she was an elementary school teacher, I decided to compare her journey to going back to college.

She would sign up for "classes" and then she would read materials and do assignments to complete the requirements. In her program, every 10 pounds would count as one class, and after she finished ten classes, she would have earned her degree.

Sara loved this idea and it gave her hope that she could lose the weight. By focusing on the small project of 10 pounds at a time, she completed all of the "classes" and was successful in reaching her goal.

Now goals

If you can't seem to stick with your exercise or weight-loss program, throw out your lofty plans and start at a simpler level. Instead of aiming for the sky, plan some *now* goals or simple steps you can take today.

Now goals begin with the words, "Today I will..." followed by an action you can easily do. Each goal should be a single item that allows you to measure whether or not you've completed it. Pick things that are simple to follow through on, then write them down or create a mental list of your goals. Here are a few examples.

Today, I will…
- Get my exercise shoes out of the closet.
- Eat an apple for my afternoon snack.
- Walk up and down one flight of stairs.
- Bring my lunch instead of going for fast food.
- Track my food intake for my evening meal.

At the end of the day, you will have either done these things or not done them. If you missed some, put them on a *now* list for tomorrow.

Over time, gradually increase what you're doing. But always keep your efforts at a realistic level. Any time you start hating your activity, take it back to a point that feels more comfortable.

It may take a year before you walk a mile or climb three flights of stairs. But rather than burn out and quit because you hate exercise, small *now* goals will help you stick with your efforts. And that's the key to achieving your big goals.

TODAY

- Create three *now* goals. Begin each one with "Today I will…"

- Write them down, then put up sticky notes as reminders.

- At the end of the day, check off the ones you've accomplished.

❧ DAY 9 ❧
When to use Plan B

Julie was upset about her social life. She said, "Every event in my schedule has food attached to it, so I end up going off my program. I get right back on the next day, but something else always pops up and there I go again!"

The fact that you are on a diet doesn't prevent others from having parties or eating dessert. So how can you have a social life and still lose weight?

Weight-Loss Plan A

Instead of sacrificing your diet for every social event, come up with a strategy for combining these two areas of your life. Begin by spelling out exactly what you do on your ideal program.

Then write down your food plan based on the number of points or calories you're aiming for most of the time. Add your exercise goals, such as a daily twenty-minute walk. All of this is your *Plan A*.

Weight-Loss Plan B

Now check what's on your calendar over the next few weeks and note the events that include food. Do you have an important party or a business trip coming up? What about your child's recital or the monthly book club or poker night?

Instead of "hoping for the best" when you head out the door, create a strategy for each of these activities. Consider how to widen your diet boundaries but stay close to your program goals. This contingency approach becomes your *Plan B.*

Assume that most of the time, you'll follow Plan A, but in situations where your diet feels too rigid, move to Plan B. For example, to use Plan A at a birthday party, you might arrive late and swap your usual beverage for a diet drink. But you can also switch to Plan B, where you enjoy one glass of wine or a small piece of cake.

Where is Plan C?

Here's the secret to having a great social life at the same time you're managing your weight. There is no Plan C! That means you don't have the option of taking the weekend off or ignoring your diet for an evening party.

With social events, always attempt to stick with either Plan A or your contingency approach, Plan B. Whenever you're tempted to skip your program, remind yourself, *there is no Plan C!*

TODAY

- Create and record a Plan A that you will follow most of the time.

- Widen the boundaries and create an optional Plan B.

- In your notebook, write the words, "There is no Plan C!"

❧ DAY 10 ❧
Do it in the fear

As I stood at the doorway of the classroom, I realized I didn't have enough courage to go in. I thought, "I'm scared to death! I don't think I can do it."

It had been fourteen years since I'd been a student. And while I was determined to follow through with my plan of getting a master's degree, I couldn't seem to make myself enter the room.

As I stood there, I remembered a mentor who told me, "When you face a scary situation, build your courage and *do it in the fear.*" With that image in mind, I walked in, slid into a chair and arranged my books on the table. Over the next two years, that same courage helped me stay in school and complete the degree.

Building courage

During my difficult recovery from breast cancer in 2010, I went on an adventure tour that included riding a zip line thousands of feet above the ground. As I stood on the platform, strapped into the zip-line harness that would carry me across a huge valley, I felt total panic. Then I remembered to reach for my courage and do it in the fear. So I jumped off the platform and successfully rode the line to the other side.

Courage represents a critical tool in your efforts to stay on a diet or conquer emotional eating. But unlike some new food plan or exercise routine, you can't pack courage neatly into a self-help book. Instead, you have to build it yourself and create ways to use it in your day.

Twenty seconds is enough

In the movie *We Bought a Zoo*, Benjamin Mee tells his son, "Sometimes all you need is twenty seconds of insane courage. Literally, twenty seconds of just embarrassing bravery. And I promise you, something great will come of it."

Courage starts with the words you say to yourself. When you face a tough time, remind yourself to reach for your courage and *do it in the fear*. Then spend twenty seconds being strong against the challenge you are facing.

Over time, the courage you find inside will grow and flourish. Eventually, it becomes the rock that holds you up and keeps you on the path to success.

TODAY

- Recall a time when fear took over your thoughts. Write it in your notebook.

- What did you do to get past the fear? Make a list of steps you took.

- Identify places in your life now where you can "do it in the fear."

DAYS 1–10 COMPLETED!

You've come this far in your 100 days...

Don't stop now. If you're struggling to stick with it, push yourself to finish *one more day*. You'll immediately be another day closer to achieving your weight-loss goals.

Just do one more day!

❧ DAYS 11–20 ❧

BUILD ON SUCCESS

❧ DAY 11 ❧
Never give up

You've started a new program, found a great place to exercise, joined a group or even started working with a life coach. *This time*, you are sure it's going to work! But then you slip up, and suddenly you feel frustrated and discouraged, just like every other time you've done this.

Now what? Do you search for a new program or a different diet book? Or just quit and go back to your old patterns? If you quit now, will it be easier at a later time, such as a year from now? And you know that once you stop a weight-loss plan, it's really hard to restart or come back to it.

Weight-loss success comes from sticking with it and not giving up, even after starting over many times. So instead of quitting, look for ways to reboot your efforts and keep at it.

The magic attempt

When people decide to stop smoking, on average, it takes quitting ten times before they become a non-smoker. Since that's the average, it means some people are successful after one try while for others, it may take twenty tries. But here's the secret. Smokers never know which attempt is the magic one that will make them successful with quitting.

In the same way, you don't know which of your weight-loss attempts will be the one that sticks. So even if you've lost weight many times in the past, your successful attempt might be right around the corner.

The value of repetition

When you don't use a particular area of your brain, it atrophies. To revive it and make it work effectively again involves repetition. So to stay on your program, you need to follow a behavior pattern consistently, day after day.

Even though research says it takes 21 days to build a habit, you can create new brain patterns a lot faster than that. All it takes is doing the behavior for three days in a row. By the third day, repetition will start to change your brain responses and will make the behavior stick.

Even during times when you struggle, never give up! Just do healthy behaviors for three days, and you'll be back on track.

TODAY

- Identify situations or events that might cause you to give up on losing weight.

- Create a phrase to remind yourself that *this* attempt might be the one that's successful.

- Build repetition by staying on your plan for three days. Then do it for another three days. Record your success.

ഐ DAY 12 ഏ
Success somewhere

When you first start a new diet, you feel strong and motivated. You are absolutely determined to reach your goal. But real life didn't change just because you went on a diet. People still bring cookies to work and invite you to birthday parties or happy hour. Others entice you to share a dessert. And eventually, you start to weaken.

Perhaps you get tired of planning and recording. Or you get sidetracked by stress, fatigue or work challenges. Next thing you know, you give in to temptation and eat six cookies or have a couple glasses of wine.

When everything goes wrong

When you get overwhelmed in life, it can seem like everything goes wrong at the same time. Because work has been crazy for weeks, your exercise plan falls apart. And your house is a disaster so you keep ordering pizza because you can't get to the grocery store. Maybe on top of everything else, your car breaks down and you don't know where you'll get the money to fix it.

During times like this, don't assume you need to fix all areas of your life at once. You just need to get *one* thing to work. From that tiny success, your energy will overflow into other areas, helping you improve them as well.

To make progress in *one* area of your life, choose a place to start and pick out one task you know you can accomplish. For example, maybe you could get back to your exercise program by doing a ten-minute walk after you get home from work.

That small success motivates you to eat something healthy for dinner. Suddenly you feel stronger about planning changes at work that will help cut your stress.

The power of *one* success

Any time you have a day when nothing goes right, simply break the pattern. Choose one small activity or task you know you can do well—then do it. It might be as simple as clearing off the kitchen counter. Once you finish, commend yourself mentally, then move on to another goal.

Each time you successfully complete a task, you reinforce a belief that you can do more. After you achieve a few small successes, you will find it easier to sustain momentum with your other goals.

TODAY

- Think about *one* thing you can do today that matches your goals.

- Write it down and post a note on your refrigerator or computer screen.

- When you've finished that *one* thing, celebrate having success somewhere.

◈ DAY 13 ◈
Get some passion

Passion! What a strange word for a weight-loss program. If you're struggling with motivation, passion is the last thing on your mind. But passion and motivation go hand in hand. When you feel one, you'll notice the other as well.

Just like motivation, passion doesn't appear out of the blue. It's something you train yourself to feel. Whether your goal is losing weight or maintaining your current weight, once you build more passion in these areas, you'll be amazed at how it affects your success.

Think about places where you need more passion. Maybe you're discouraged because you ate too much during a recent vacation or at a family reunion. Or maybe you hate exercise and can't get yourself out the door for a walk. Perhaps you feel overwhelmed because you need to lose a lot of weight and don't know where to start.

Wouldn't it be great to have passion instead of discouragement in all of these areas? So how do you find passion? The answer is… you don't! You create it. Passion comes as a result of giving extra focus and attention to specific areas in your life.

Make this your passion week

Creating passion requires that you live from a place of energy and confidence, not fear and insecurity. To build passion, you have to fire up your own actions and, in some areas, push yourself a little harder. Like a tiny spark that creates a roaring fire, passion grows when you give it fuel. The more you focus on it, the stronger it becomes.

Maybe you yearn for a new job or a fresh relationship. Perhaps you want to build stronger connections with your children or spouse. You can use the passion theme for your job, your family, even your pets.

Pick one specific area, then pour some passion into it. Give that goal extra attention, energy, focus and love. You'll be amazed at how differently you'll feel about this area of your life. You will also have deepened your commitment to your program just by focusing harder on your goal.

Creating passion begins with taking action. Even the smallest micro movement can get you unstuck and moving toward a renewed sense of hope and accomplishment.

TODAY

- Choose one area of your life that you'd like to improve. Write it down and plan to create some passion for it.

- For the entire day, give this area extra attention, energy and focus.

- At the end of the day, notice the difference in your actions. Record this in your notebook.

❧ DAY 14 ❧
Ditch the parent

When Susie stopped at her mom's home after work, she gave in to her cravings and ate two large brownies. She told me, "I gave myself permission to eat them, so I figured it was OK."

Does this sound familiar? In order to justify eating something that's not on your diet, you simply give yourself permission to have a slip-up. You tell yourself, "You've been a very good child, so I'll give you permission to eat that wonderful treat."

Giving yourself permission to eat means you're taking a parental approach to your behaviors. The parent said you couldn't have a brownie, but you rebelled and gave yourself permission. Of course, now you're in trouble and you can't seem to get back into the good graces of the parent part of your brain.

I find it interesting that we rarely use the word *permission* in other areas of life. Do you give yourself permission to take a bathroom break or to drive fast? This probably never crosses your mind.

Permission to eat is usually a shame-based action rather than a carefully pondered intention. Shame results from setting up a controversy between *good* and *bad* behavior. When you eliminate the use of these words, you don't get pulled into a mental battle, and shame doesn't have any reason to show up.

Time to grow up

Maybe you've tried giving yourself permission to eat certain foods because that's supposed to stop cravings. But this still assumes that, if you are a strong, demanding parent, you will not misbehave by eating.

Think about this question. When was the last time you gave yourself permission *not* to eat a brownie? Usually, the word *permission* never crosses your mind. So let go of using it to describe why you ate a brownie or other foods not on your diet.

Instead of giving yourself permission, refer to the *choices* you make in your life. For example, if you eat an unplanned cookie, tell yourself, "I chose to eat that."

It's time to take back your power around food. When you're in charge of your life, you don't have to worry about permission to eat. Use language that supports your power, not a bossy, parental approach toward food and eating.

TODAY

- Identify and record a recent time when you ate a cookie or other treat.

- Write the words, "I chose to eat..." and add the food you listed above.

- Each time you eat something today, tell yourself, "I'm choosing to eat this." Write a note about how that felt.

✎ DAY 15 ✎
Beat myself up

I was doing great all week. Then my mom made my favorite layer cake and I ate two pieces. But I didn't beat myself up about it!"

That famous line, "I didn't beat myself up," ranks toward the top of my list of stupid things dieters say. I know it's supposed to replace the negative self-talk about falling off your diet. But when you proclaim, "I didn't beat myself up," you are simply ignoring your behavior.

The fact that you didn't scold yourself is certainly healthier for your self-esteem. But it also admits that you didn't learn anything. It's sort of like getting a failing grade at school but not contemplating how to study better for the next exam.

If you are determined to be successful in your weight-management efforts, ignoring your slip-ups is not a good idea. Instead, start taking a look at what you learned or still need to learn.

Next time you have a slip-up, ask yourself three questions:

1. What happened? Where was the break in my plan or the point when I let up and ignored my goals?

2. What was going on? Was I stressed? Lonely? Anxious? Was I simply tired of monitoring everything I eat?

3. What did I learn? How can I recognize this type of event or emotional need and protect myself better when it comes up again?

Look at what you've learned

Suppose you went to visit your mother and gave in to the chocolate cake. Afterward, you say to yourself, "OK, I ate two pieces of cake at my mom's house. Even though she means well, my mother still has the ability to irritate me with her comments. I've learned that I need to be more prepared next time I see her. Perhaps I could take a walk to let go of my stress before I arrive at her house."

If you don't learn anything from your eating mistake, you'll probably keep repeating the behavior. Rather than ignoring a slip-up and hoping for the best, put your foot down firmly. Tell yourself, "That was unfortunate. It was not what I'd planned. And here's what I've learned…" Then live in confidence that you'll be stronger in the future.

TODAY

- Think about a recent time when you ate snacks or desserts you hadn't planned on eating.

- Answer the three questions: what happened, what was going on, what did I learn?

- Record your answers, then lay out a plan for managing this situation better in the future.

✎ DAY 16 ❧

Compulsive or impulsive eating?

Do you ever start eating in the morning and keep nibbling the rest of the day? Or do you take a few bites of leftover cake, then feel like you can't stop so you eat it all? Perhaps you have times when you feel out of control and eat everything in sight.

If these behaviors sound familiar, you may have decided you are a *compulsive overeater.* In truth, you probably don't fit the definition at all. The word *compulsive* refers to an uncontrolled, urgent desire that usually can't be stopped voluntarily.

By that definition, your eating patterns are not compulsive. Instead, you probably are an *impulsive* overeater. If you've ever become angry enough to throw something against the wall or slam your fist on the table, you understand impulsive behaviors.

Often, impulsive eating involves reaching for food to fix or avoid something in your life. For example, when you experience an emotion you don't like, such as grief, on impulse you eat to make that feeling go away.

Triggers such as seeing or smelling food can also prompt an impulsive eating response. Or you might do impulsive eating when you feel stressed, frustrated or sad. But, unlike compulsive behaviors, you *can* stop. To do this, you need to train yourself to manage impulses differently around food. For example, you could respond to stress by taking a walk instead of grabbing something to eat.

The seven-minute solution

Addictions counseling teaches that a craving rarely lasts longer than seven minutes. So by forcing yourself to avoid food for that long, you can usually overcome continuous eating. For example, if you get hooked into eating chips, cookie dough or some other type of snack, simply force yourself to take a seven-minute break from the food.

Follow these three steps:

1. Say to yourself, "Of course I can stop eating this." Then set a timer or alarm for seven minutes.
2. Move away from the food. Go into another room or get outdoors. Distract yourself in some way.
3. For the next seven minutes, do something active and positive.

You'll be amazed how easily you can stop an eating frenzy. When you interrupt the pattern by taking a seven-minute break, you'll have managed your impulsive eating.

TODAY

- Watch for a time today when you feel tempted to eat something not on your plan.

- For seven minutes, stay away from the food. Do something positive during this time.

- Write a note in your journal about what you did and then describe how this worked.

⤺ DAY 17 ⤻
Do I really care?

Using a flower such as a daisy, you can pull off one petal at a time while saying the two phrases, "He loves me; he loves me not." Whichever one you say as you remove the last petal provides the answer to your love life.

Sometimes your weight-loss efforts might feel as random as this flower petal game. The only difference is that you're trying to decide whether you care or don't care about losing weight.

Some days, you are certain that you care. Then a few days later, you decide to skip your workout and eat whatever you want. You just pulled out the *I don't care* petal.

But what if that petal comes up a lot? Maybe you *care* during the week, but *don't care* on weekends. Unfortunately, the *don't care* days can undo the progress you made on the days you did care. Eventually, weeks or even months can go by without any progress on losing weight.

Something is affecting you

Not sticking with your diet plan doesn't always mean you don't care. Instead, it's usually a sign that something else requires your attention.

Try to identify things that are demanding your energy and focus right now. Perhaps you're stressed and overworked. Or maybe you're dreading a holiday season filled with bored kids, travel or out-of-town guests.

Once you label what's affecting your ability to care, create a plan for managing things better. Consider ways to get more rest, relax more or decrease the stress from life and family demands.

How many days do you want to care?

Each morning, ask yourself, "Is this a day when I *care* or one when I *don't care*?" Once you label it as a day that you care, live that way all day.

Even if you're tired or not feeling motivated, remind yourself you *do* care. Then head for your workout even if you don't feel like it. When you're tempted to reach for a bag of cookies, say, "No! This is a day that I *care*, so I won't eat that." Because deep inside, you really *do* care.

TODAY

- Make a sign that says, "I do care." Post it where you can see it easily or carry it inside your pocket or purse.

- Write down ways you will demonstrate that you care today. Then eat your healthy meals, take your walk and use positive self-talk to prove that you care.

- At the end of the day, notice the difference in your actions. Record this in your notebook.

❧ DAY 18 ❧

I know what works

In the children's story, *The Wizard of Oz*, a young farm girl named Dorothy travels down a yellow brick road in search of a way to get back to her home in Kansas. During her adventure, she meets several unusual characters who become part of the journey.

These delightful storybook friends are all seeking a piece of life they believe will give them true happiness. Yet as we follow them on their travels, we soon realize they already have what they are looking for. They simply aren't able to recognize and appreciate their unique gifts.

In a similar way, you may think you are lacking something vital to your success. Maybe you believe you can't lose weight or stop emotional eating until you've found the ideal book or discovered the perfect diet plan.

Or perhaps you've concluded you don't have enough self-discipline or you can't resist certain foods. But like the characters in Dorothy's story, you already have the solution to being successful.

Study what went wrong

When you've lost weight, then gained it all back, it's easy to blame the diet. But to get the real answer, study the time between when you were at your goal weight and when you had regained weight. What changed? Did you let go of your exercise program? Drink more alcohol and eat more desserts? Stop caring?

You probably know what causes you to fall off the diet wagon—things such as emotional eating or loss of motivation. Maybe your demanding schedule or a challenging job drains your time and energy. When you can recognize the things that cause you to stumble, you can take steps to change the patterns.

Go back to what works

Think about times when you've successfully lost or maintained your weight in the past. What did you do, and how did you make it work? Did you cook more meals? Go to the gym? Walk your dog every day? Perhaps you kept a journal, went to meetings or met with a diet counselor.

Sometimes new and fresh ideas can boost your motivation. But don't lose sight of what you already know. Pull out the tools that have worked for you in the past and start using them again.

TODAY

- Make a list of tools or actions that worked great for you in the past.

- Choose one of these things that will still work for you. Write it down.

- Put that tool into your day and use it to stay on your plan. Record how this went.

⟡ DAY 19 ⟡
Hope—the secret word

Ellen sank into my office chair and let out a huge sigh. "I'm so discouraged," she said. "I've been working on my weight for so long, and I can't seem to get anywhere. Right now, I don't think I'll ever reach my goal. I feel so hopeless!"

"Let's start with your story," I said. "Tell me about your weight-loss journey."

"It's a long one," she began. "Right now, I need to lose at least 100 pounds. And over the years, I've tried everything from diet books to weekly meetings, and even meal-replacement plans. Each time, I lose about 25 or 30 pounds, but then something happens and my motivation goes away. Within a short time, I always gain it all back. I just don't know if I can do this anymore!"

The secret word

Many of you have a story similar to Ellen's. Whether you need to lose 20 pounds or 200 pounds, the pattern she described can be devastating.

When it comes to losing weight or maintaining long-term, do you know the top predictor of success? It's not a new diet book, going to a different program or finding the right group leader. It's having *hope*.

Research shows that one of the most common causes of regaining weight is sliding into discouragement. When this happens, you lose motivation, and eventually you lose hope that you'll ever be successful.

Even when it seems like you'll never reach your goals, *hope* will move you forward and sustain your efforts day after day. Here are three things hope can do for you:

1. Hope releases you from your past. Instead of assuming you'll repeat the lose/regain pattern, hope fuels a belief that you *can* be successful with your goals.

2. Hope motivates you to keep going in spite of tough times. It helps you bounce back after a day of overeating or skipping exercise. It's what pushes you to get back up instead of giving up.

3. Hope activates you. It becomes the fuel that keeps you going, even when the odds are against you. Hope encourages you to take steps toward your goals every day, even when it feels impossible to reach them.

TODAY

*   How hopeful do you feel right now? A lot, some, a little or not at all? Write it down.

*   Describe recent times when you've lost hope, including what caused this to happen.

*   Identify one step you can take today to build a sense of hope and optimism.

❧ DAY 20 ❧
Rebuild your hope

If your sense of hope has slipped away, you may need to work on rebuilding it. Hope is more than just an emotion you feel. It's a *state of being* you create by your thoughts, your beliefs and your actions. Regardless of personality style or life history, almost anyone can learn to have hope.

Listen to your *hope voice*

We all have little voices inside our heads, constantly giving us all kinds of advice. Be sure to pay attention to which voices you are listening to. Recognize the one that whines about your failure or reminds you about your discouragement. Then consciously push the button that will shut that voice off.

You may have to search a bit, but find your voice of hope and make it stronger. Start with a tiny glow of light, then nurture your hope day by day until it feels like a powerful beacon. Here are three ways to work on this and build a stronger sense of hope.

1. Recharge your batteries

Take a quick look at your current life issues. Then make a list of what drains you and what fuels you. Of course, you probably can't eliminate all the things that drain you. But you can push yourself to focus on the ones that refuel you and help keep you moving toward your goals.

2. Raise your expectations

Do this with your life as well as your weight-loss plan. Build a belief that reaching your goal is possible and that your current efforts will work. If you stay consistent with it, any diet or exercise plan will bring results. So hold onto a sense of hope, that of course, you will be successful.

3. Look ahead, not back

The first lesson in *100 Days of Weight Loss* proclaims that your past does not determine your future. Do you have a long list of programs you've already tried? So what? That has nothing to do with your ability to be successful now.

Let go of the *past* and remind yourself that now you are in a different place with new tools that will propel you forward. Listen to your *hope voice* often and train it to give you words of love and encouragement every single day!

TODAY

- Identify things your negative voice tells you. For example, "I never stay on a plan."

- Reframe those thoughts by writing, "That's not true... I can overcome that."

- Create a powerful statement to use as your *hope voice*. For example, "Of course I can do this!"

43

DAYS 11–20 COMPLETED!

You've come this far in your 100 days...

Don't stop now. If you're struggling to stick with it, push yourself to finish *one more day*. You'll immediately be another day closer to achieving your weight-loss goals.

Just do one more day!

❧ DAYS 21–30 ❧

KEEP FOOD WHERE IT BELONGS

Day 21   The couch is calling

Day 22   When not to eat dinner

Day 23   Food and nurturing

Day 24   Planning to overeat

Day 25   After the party's over

Day 26   Vacations and reunions

Day 27   Skip it or savor it

Day 28   Get your money's worth

Day 29   Healthy day hat

Day 30   Feel blessed

∽ DAY 21 ∾
The couch is calling

As I settled into a booth at the coffee shop, a cheerful voice announced, "Good morning! My name is Lori and I'll be serving you today."

And she did! Lori filled my coffee cup again and again while also taking care of other customers in the busy restaurant. Finally I commented, "You sure are running a lot. You must get really tired."

Her response was quick. "Yes, I do. And with all of this work, you'd think I'd be skinny. But for some reason, I never lose a pound!"

As we chatted, Lori confessed that, when she got home from work, she would usually lie on the couch to rest before planning her evening. Of course, once she was on the couch, it felt impossible to get back off the couch. So instead of exercising, she just stayed there.

"What am I doing wrong?" she asked. "Why am I not losing anything?" The answer was simple. Lori was operating on a common misconception about what it takes to drop some pounds.

It's not exercise

Unfortunately, being on your feet all day doesn't energize you or help you lose weight. It just makes you tired. First of all, your body adapts to the activity level and no longer views it as a challenge to your system. Secondly, those start and stop movements don't build muscle or raise your heart rate enough to result in weight loss.

Any time you move your body, it's still better than not moving it. But to actually lose weight, you need activity that's more rhythmic and sustained, such as walking, biking or swimming.

I suggested to Lori that she tell herself, "I can do whatever I want, including lie on the couch, after I take a walk." Within a few weeks of her new plan, Lori reported that exercising actually gave her energy instead of making her more tired. She said, "It's amazing! I was so sure that I'd be way too tired to do this. But I reminded myself that I only had to do a short walk. It worked every time, and it did make me feel better."

TODAY

- Create a weekly exercise plan to include the type of activity, length of time and which days you will exercise.

- Plan ways to get past the barriers, such as fatigue, schedule or stress, that would prevent you from exercising.

- Record your exercise activity every day for at least a week. Note how you feel as a result of more activity.

✎ DAY 22 ❧

When not to eat dinner

Lori, the waitress from yesterday's lesson, was frustrated with her weight-loss plan. She said, "Most days, I'm really good when I'm at work. In fact, lots of times I don't eat anything during the day, hoping that will work like a diet. Of course, by the time I get home, I'm so hungry that I grab whatever's handy and usually nibble on junk food the rest of the evening."

Unfortunately, not eating all day doesn't drop the pounds. Many experts believe that when you avoid eating during the day, your body slows down in response to the famine. Later, your body will store some of what you take in during the evening because it anticipates there may be a food shortage again the next day.

In Lori's case, her diet was actually causing her to overeat. To fix her problem with junk food in the evening, I suggested Lori follow these steps:

1. Use the five-hour rule

Anytime you go longer than five hours between eating, you are likely to do three things: eat too much, make poor food choices and not care. By dividing her calories out over the day, Lori could avoid being overly hungry once she got home.

2. Eat mini-meals

I suggested to Lori that instead of assuming she can't eat right because she doesn't have time for a meal, she come up with healthy snacks that could serve as mini-meals throughout her busy days. Her list included mozzarella cheese sticks, small cartons of yogurt, protein food bars and even containers of applesauce for times when fruit would take too much time or effort.

3. Don't eat dinner right away

Plan to build in a transition between work and dinner so you'll feel more like making a healthy meal. Lori decided to first take her walk, then eat a snack to manage her hunger and renew her energy.

This idea works even if you have a family clamoring for food. If your own tank is empty, you aren't going to manage your fuel needs very well. An afternoon snack provides a great transition, but plan for it so you have healthy options. Even sitting a few minutes with a cup of tea or a cold drink will help you manage your evening better.

TODAY

- Identify places in your day where you might go longer than five hours between eating.

- Plan a transition between your activities of the day and your evening meal.

- Create a short list of mini meals or snacks; then stock up on supplies for them.

ॐ DAY 23 ॐ
Food and nurturing

Lori, the waitress, made great progress by changing her daily routine. But she was stuck in the pattern of nibbling on junk food all evening while she watched TV. Ever since her divorce two years ago, Lori had struggled with feeling sad and alone in the evenings. Her comment was, "Once I get home to that empty house, all I want is junk food."

What she was really saying is, "I want something that nurtures me and helps fill this empty space in my life." Of course, her ritual of TV channel surfing while mindlessly eating cookies or chips never fixed the problem. By the time she headed for bed, she usually felt bloated and disgusted. But she couldn't figure out how to fix it.

Lori's situation does not have an easy answer. You can't fix an empty life by simply eating carrots instead of potato chips. But here's a few easy steps that can help you nurture yourself instead of heading to the refrigerator for evening comfort.

Change the ritual

Although she had a couple of favorite shows, Lori realized that, many nights, she could skip watching TV entirely. On those evenings, she intentionally left the TV off and worked on an alternate activity.

Sometimes she got absorbed in an engaging novel. Other times, she worked on crafts or went shopping. Before long, she discovered that her new activities were more appealing than watching TV.

Draw on music

To fill the quiet when the TV was off, Lori began listening to her favorite music from past years. She delighted in renewing her interest in jazz and choral music. She soon learned that listening to upbeat music improved her mood as well as her energy level.

Get some input

Lori used to enjoy sewing, so one Saturday she took a quilting class. There she met a couple of women who invited her to join their monthly quilting club. Besides providing a way to pursue her new hobby, this also helped her develop some wonderful new friendships.

As a result of altering her negative patterns, Lori felt like a new person. She lost 20 pounds and improved her health as well as her energy level. But most importantly, she realized these simple changes in her life are ones she can stick with forever.

TODAY

- When are your worst times of day with food and eating issues?

- Identify at least two alternate activities you can do during this time.

- Record how this works and whether it changes your eating patterns.

∽ DAY 24 ∾
Planning to overeat

Jeremy had been through a stressful week with out-of-town travel related to his work. As he reflected on the hard week, he said, "I knew I was going to eat a bunch. It's as though I made up my mind long before I was around the food, and I couldn't figure out how to stop the train."

As we analyzed Jeremy's behavior patterns, we identified a few of the reasons for his eating struggle. He wanted a break and some relief from his stressful work. He actually knew ahead of time that he was going to go off his diet and overeat.

This often happens in response to long, hard weeks with high stress levels as well as travel or other demands. By Friday morning, you secretly begin plotting a visit to your favorite Italian restaurant, knowing that, once you get there, your boundaries will evaporate. In other words, you plan your eating binge ahead of time.

I deserve a break

Jeremy told me that he'd been very stressed and he had "too much on his plate." I laughed as he described how he got things "off his plate." He said, "I guess I overate to feel some relief from the burdens of my life."

When you've had a stressful week or month, you do deserve a break. But food doesn't have to be your break of choice. Think about other ways you can recover or feel nurtured. Even taking a walk or relaxing with a diet soda instead of a beer will help change the pattern.

Make a new plan

You wouldn't tell a police officer that you "planned to drive fast," so you don't deserve a speeding ticket. Instead, if you catch a glimpse of your speedometer creeping up, you quickly slow down and get back within the speed limit. You can do the same thing with your eating thoughts.

Recognize when you are planning to overeat and immediately slam on your mental brakes. Remind yourself that wolfing down a plate of pasta and chasing it with cheesecake isn't going to move you toward your weight-loss goals. Focus on the benefits of staying on track with your plans for healthier eating and exercise, then find a different way to give yourself a break.

TODAY

- Identify an event or situation where you might end up planning to overeat.

- Is that what you really want to do? Is it worth it? Write your answer.

- List three things you will do to prevent sliding into overeating in this situation.

✎ DAY 25 ✎
After the party's over

At her weekly family dinner, Sylvia usually stayed on her diet plan by picking at her salad and refusing dessert. But she secretly harbored lots of resentment. She felt deprived and left out when everyone else was eating lasagna and homemade pie.

She told me, "It didn't seem fair, and I guess a part of me wanted to get even with them. So after I got home, I ate everything I didn't get to eat earlier." What went wrong? Sylvia got caught in *after the party's over* syndrome.

Lots of times you may notice feeling let down or disappointed after you've made a concerted effort to eat carefully. During this letdown period, you are at high risk for overeating.

In my work, I've observed this happening a lot around holidays such as Thanksgiving. My clients would plan a detailed strategy for managing Thanksgiving dinner and they typically got through the holiday extremely well. But on the Friday after Thanksgiving, they would start eating in the morning and eat all day long, sometimes even continuing through the weekend.

After the party's over syndrome usually occurs after a period of being exceptionally competent with managing an eating event. But sometimes, while you're being so strong in the face of food temptations or social norms, you're secretly feeling insecure or unsure of yourself. Perhaps you resent the fact you can't participate in celebrating like everyone else, so you make up for it later.

Plan for after the party

The solution to this pattern involves preparing for any event by planning twice. Besides your careful thoughts on how you will handle the party or gathering, you need to add a detailed plan for the evening or the day after the event.

If you host a gathering in your home, have a plan for handling the leftovers or the empty time after guests have gone. Include ways to fill your spirit back up when you are stressed or tired from all the effort it takes to resist overeating.

The bigger the event, the more you need an afterward plan. It's all about the letdown. Just know that it's going to be there and get ahead of the game by planning for both the event and the time after it's over.

TODAY

- Identify situations where you are at risk for eating after an event is over.

- Come up with three self-care things you will routinely do to manage this.

- Create a detailed after-the-party plan for the day (or two) after the event.

✎ DAY 26 ✎
Vacation and reunions

Vacations, reunions and travel can all make it seem impossible to stay on your diet or exercise program. But "getting away from it all" doesn't mean you have to give up on managing your weight.

Start by labeling any trip or vacation as a time for taking care of yourself. Then plan in lots of activities that will make you stronger and healthier. And whether you're dancing at your high school reunion or gathering with family at holidays, remind yourself that you don't need lots of food to appreciate the good times in life.

Use these tips to manage your weight during vacations, family gatherings or reunions that challenge your ability to stay on your program.

Start with water

Drink a glass of water as soon as you wake up. The minute you finish it, label your day as being a healthy one. By meeting part of your water requirements, you've already started taking care of yourself.

Exercise daily

Begin each day with a walk or some type of exercise. Use this activity to set the tone for the day. Once you've exercised, you won't be as tempted to eat or drink in ways that will undo your efforts.

Half-off special

When you're faced with lots of food, use the concept of the half-off special. Simply eat half as much as you normally would or take half of the amount you actually want. This helps you control portions at restaurants as well as family dinners where other people put food in front of you.

Do a tasting diet

Feel free to experiment with trying new foods or enjoying desserts. But with anything that isn't part of your fuel needs for the day, have just a taste or limit yourself to two bites. Savor the food, appreciate the flavors, then walk away from the table and do something else.

Minimize the damage

Rather than dropping your good intentions once you arrive at your destination, look for ways to lower the risk of overeating. Always eat a healthy snack before showing up at an event. Or fill your wine glass with water and pretend it's a cocktail. If you do slip up, minimize the damage by stopping yourself quickly, then getting right back on track.

TODAY

- Create a vacation or reunion plan, even if those times are months away.

- Decide how you will track your actions during those events. Record your plan.

- Put your plan on a small card or in a memo on your phone so you'll have it available when you need it.

❧ DAY 27 ❧

Skip it or savor it

Bonnie admitted that she struggled a lot with snack foods. Whenever she went to a party or book club meeting, she would promise herself that she would manage the bowls of nuts and chocolate-covered pretzels, but it never worked.

She would start by having just a few snacks, but then she'd keep eating more until she'd gone way past her calorie plan. She said, "Once I start eating, I just can't seem to stop." Working on ways to manage her snack food challenge, we came up with several ideas.

Skip it entirely

Plan to always eat something before you go to a gathering. By taking care of your fuel needs, you'll be less hungry and have more stamina against food pushers.

At the event, stay as far away from the food as possible. If someone asks why you aren't eating, explain that you just finished a meal and you need to wait awhile. Then draw on tools such as postponing eating or telling yourself, "Don't even start."

Savor it

Whenever you eat snacks, be sure to savor the taste. Take very small bites and pay close attention to the flavor and texture of the food. Also, look for ways to manage the amounts you eat. For example, consider a one-inch serving of dessert. This works great with birthday cake, pies and bar cookies. Just cut off a section that's about one-inch square, then take tiny bites and savor the food.

If you enjoy small candies or nuts, eat them with a fork. Be sure you pay attention to the texture and the "mouth feel" of the snack. You'll be amazed at how this stops the pattern of constantly reaching for more.

It's not my food

Any time you want to avoid eating snacks or sweets, use the powerful line "It's not my food." Simply tell yourself that the food is for someone else, and it doesn't belong to you.

Pretend the snacks are in someone's grocery basket or on the desk of a grouchy person. Then remind yourself not to go near the food. Use inner self-talk such as, "That doesn't belong to me," or "It's not something for me to eat." Even repeating the simple line "Not my food" can help you avoid the temptation of snacks.

TODAY

- Watch for situations where sweets or snack foods tempt you.

- Each time, decide whether to skip the food or savor it. Record your experiences.

- Intentionally label something as "Not my food." Describe how this worked.

❧ DAY 28 ❧
Get your money's worth

Don was a volume eater. He grew up on a farm where family members worked long, hard hours and were rewarded with huge home-cooked meals. His love of food stayed with him, and large meals always reminded him of those good days on the farm.

He said, "Growing up, my father told us to be sure we got our money's worth at restaurants. I've always been proud of the fact that no restaurant buffet has ever made money off me." Unfortunately, Don's love of big meals contributed to his becoming extremely overweight. But he couldn't bear the thought of giving up large servings.

Don had two issues to overcome. Eating large amounts was easy to change because he began tracking his meals and monitoring his calorie intake. But he struggled at restaurants because of the old message from his father. So we had to figure out how to change the way he defined getting his money's worth of food.

Create a new message

Whenever you go to a restaurant, you anticipate spending a certain amount of money to enjoy a meal and good conversation without having to cook or wash dishes. From the time you order your meal, you've made a decision. You are going pay a set amount of money for that dining experience.

How much food do you have to eat before you've accomplished those goals? The answer is, "Whenever you've

eaten enough to fuel your body." Once you have completed
what you came for, you got your money's worth.

Don decided that when he planned to eat out, he would
figure out ahead of time how much he would spend on his
meal. For that money, he would anticipate enjoying his food
as well as the company of the people he was with. And that
became how he would define getting his money's worth.

Learn to measure the value of eating out by the flavors
of the food and the quality of the experience, not the food
volume. Eating more doesn't increase the value you're getting.
In fact, it can make the event less enjoyable because you
become unhappy about eating too much.

TODAY

- Make a list of what you want at restaurants,
  such as fuel for your body, tasty food and
  great conversation.

- Plan a restaurant meal for sometime soon
  and decide how much you will spend.

- At the restaurant, notice when you've
  gotten the things on your list, then stop
  eating at that point. Record whether you
  got your money's worth.

∾ DAY 29 ∾
Healthy day hat

Tanya was in a panic! After maintaining her weight for months, she had started overeating again. She said. "I'm scared I'll start gaining weight back. How do I stop this quickly?"

"First of all," I began, "I want you to know that you are normal. Many people do great for a long time, then suddenly feel like they're going backward. Sometimes you can fix it simply by changing the way you see yourself."

When you notice you're slipping back into old patterns, here's a great solution. Each morning, pretend you put on a healthy day hat. You could even put on a real hat if you wish. Then do these five things that help you label the day as being a healthy one.

1. The magic glass of water

Each morning, start the day by drinking a glass of water. (That's one down already.) This immediately demonstrates that it's a healthy day.

2. One healthy meal

Eat a specific breakfast that you can count on as being healthy. Consider eggs and toast, or maybe oatmeal and fruit. After you've eaten one healthy meal, you're more likely to make good choices for the other meals in your day.

3. Do a little bit of exercise

Even a short walk or a few minutes on a treadmill will work. I like the idea of pushing yourself to do ten minutes. After that, you can stay with it and keep going or quit for the day. Either way, you'll feel like a success.

4. Eliminate the food fix

Every time you head for the refrigerator or cupboard, remind yourself that your emotional needs, such as feeling anxious or stressed, are not going to be fixed by eating. Sure, it's kind of soothing, but in the long run, you'll just be upset and feel worse.

5. Instant nurturing

Make a short list of things that will calm or nurture you, such as sitting down with a cup of tea and forcing yourself to slow down a bit. Do at least one thing from your list each day.

By hanging the "Healthy Day" sign over your head each morning, you'll be inspired to stay with your diet or maintenance program successfully the rest of the day.

TODAY

- In your notebook or computer document, write the words "Today is a healthy day."

- Create a list of several things you will include in your plan today.

- At the end of the day, check off the ones you accomplished. Celebrate that it was a healthy day.

∽ DAY 30 ∾
Feel blessed

"Needing therapy?" he asked quietly as he watched me pull out the flour, sugar and chocolate chips. "Just a little," I replied. My husband has learned that when I start baking, there's usually something else going on.

As I contemplated why I had a sudden urge to make chocolate chip cookies, I realized I was not happy with December. No matter how many times I hear the song, "It's the most wonderful time of the year," I will never believe that. Instead, I think it's a hard month, filled with stress, worry and disappointment.

For many people, December is a month plagued by sadness and difficult emotions. The image of cozy family gatherings around a holiday tree is often shattered by the reality of divorce, job loss or financial problems. It also includes loved ones who are ill or no longer with us.

December typically brings lots of food temptations with parties, desserts and food gifts. But even if December (or any difficult time for you) is months away, you can begin planning how to handle it in healthier ways.

Do extreme self-care

To practice managing any type of holiday, set a goal of doing extreme self-care over the weeks ahead. For a few minutes each day, make time for yourself and your own needs. Look for ways to feel calm, peaceful and even nurtured during the demanding times.

Sip a cup of tea while sitting in your dining room or in a cozy chair by the fireplace. Put on some soothing music, light a candle and take a break from your life challenges. A few minutes of quiet reflection can do wonders for your inner spirit.

Choose to feel blessed

Rather than chase the elusive feelings of happiness, pay attention to areas where you feel blessed. Appreciate the people you love, be grateful for the good things around you, and let others know you are feeling blessed.

For me, this is a great reminder for the month of December as well as any time I feel overwhelmed by life challenges. When I feel irritated with the holiday music, I start reciting the ways that I'm blessed. It doesn't change the realities of December, but it sure cuts down on baking cookies for therapy.

TODAY

- Create a one-day plan for extreme self-care. Include non-food things that feel nurturing.

- Do each of the things on your list, and record how it felt to take extra care of yourself.

- Write a list of ways you are blessed right now. Read your list several times today.

DAYS 21–30 COMPLETED!

You've come this far in your 100 days...

Don't stop now. If you're struggling to stick with it, push yourself to finish *one more day*. You'll immediately be another day closer to achieving your weight-loss goals.

Just do one more day!

❧ DAYS 31–40 ❧

SUSTAIN MOTIVATION

∽ DAY 31 ∾
Restore yourself

When he opened the creaky door of the old farm garage, David could hardly believe his eyes. Covered in dust sat a red 1968 Mustang. The frame was rusted along the bottom, and dents marred the hood and the sides. The interior was awful with torn seats and a musty odor.

"What a beauty!" David exclaimed. "To most people, this car looks like junk. But it just needs to be restored. I'll tow it to my shop and by the end of the year, it will be transformed into a classic. When I take it on the road, it may not perform like a Mustang of today. But it will be solid and strong, and it will take me where I want to go."

David bought the Mustang and worked on it every day. A year later, he eased it out of his garage and headed down the road, singing at the top of his lungs. He had restored his dream car.

Perhaps you feel like that old Mustang—rusted, tired, overweight or discouraged. But just like David, you can find energy and fix your body size by working on a restoration project.

How to restore yourself

1. Make a list of areas you want to restore. Your list might include your weight, eating patterns, exercise, cooking, sewing or crafts, and friendships or groups.

2. Determine what's needed for restoring each area. Some things will be simple and quick, such as cooking healthier

meals or pulling out a favorite recipe book. Others will require more planning, preparation or learning.

3. Work on the list a little each day. You can't restore all of your projects at the same time. So get realistic and choose carefully what you want to focus on.

Start right away

If you keep postponing your restoration project, a year from now nothing will have changed. So get going. Every day, work on restoring a tiny bit of your life. As the months go by, you'll be able to see a lot more of your original structure, beauty and value.

Even when it's hard, keep your vision clear and focused. Some parts will be easy to rebuild, others quite difficult. But eventually your efforts will pay off as you restore and appreciate your life.

TODAY

- Write a list of areas you'd like to restore in your life.

- For each item, write down one thing that will help you begin restoring it.

- Choose one goal and take action on it today. Record what you did.

ഽ DAY 32 ൫
Make exercise work

Once the couch becomes more attractive than lacing up your exercise shoes, you're in big trouble. Motivation goes into hiding and your frequent thoughts that today you'll get back on track do no good whatsoever.

We all know that exercise is necessary, but that's not enough to keep us on a plan. Instead, most of us have times when we become exercise dropouts. Changing a few rules about your exercise program might help you stay with it.

You don't need to love it

You've probably heard that if you find a type of exercise you love, your struggles will disappear. For many of us, that isn't ever going to happen. That's like thinking that if you love parenting, your kids will never get on your nerves. Better advice is to love your children, and learn how to be patient on days you don't love parenting.

With exercise, focus on loving your body and taking care of it. Then work on using exercise as a tool to accomplish your goals.

You don't need an hour every day

If you're overweight or out of shape, pushing for this level of exercise just doesn't make sense. Not only will it be hard on your joints, it will also make you so tired you won't care about getting healthy and you'll simply quit.

Instead, set a goal of doing something every day. Take a ten-minute walk or ride your bike around the block. Over time, you can gradually increase your exercise amount. And if you get to the point where you like working out for an hour every day, that's fine. If not, do what I do—celebrate any day that you move your body for twenty or thirty minutes.

Give it time

Quit looking in the mirror to see if your stomach has changed by a quarter of an inch. It takes time to re-shape a lumpy body. Rather than setting your sights on being the poster child for bodybuilding, do the types of exercise that work for you.

What's most important is that you move versus not move. So keep working on your exercise program, even if it's small. Over time, the results will show, and you'll know it was all worth the effort.

TODAY

- Write down the smallest amount of exercise you could do most days.

- Plan how you will put that in place today.

- Record what you did and how it felt to have a small, realistic goal.

❧ DAY 33 ❧
Create some joy

Once in a while, I feel really grouchy. I don't have any big reason for this—maybe it's the weather or not enough sleep or a backache. I could really use some nurturing or a bit of encouragement.

But there's no one to give me attention or kindness when I need it. People around me are concerned about their own lives and don't even notice my sad mood or my frustration. As a result, I've learned that I have to take care of my own needs for nurturing.

What do you love?

Here's a great exercise for helping you boost your spirits and create some joy. Take a few minutes to think about what you love. Consider everything that energizes you, gives you joy or fills you with delight.

Now take out a piece of paper and write the words "What I Love" at the top of the page. Then list everything you can think of that matches that description. Include people, activities and pets as well as meaningful things such as sunsets or green grass.

You might include events such as concerts, plays and vacations. Perhaps you love sports or crafts or reading. Be sure to add soothing, relaxing things such as a warm bath, massage or yoga. If you find encouragement through online sites such as Pinterest, add some of your favorite motivational phrases to your list.

Don't spend a long time thinking about this—simply write down everything you consider nurturing, even if some of the items are not always available or accessible.

The six-month check

Once you've completed your list, put a check mark next to anything you haven't done, seen or appreciated in the past six months. Use these marks to identify all the nurturing activities you've lost touch with or forgotten about.

For me, playing my piano and singing always show up on my six-month list. It's a shame too, because music always nurtures and comforts me, especially during really hard times. I also love to go dancing and usually discover it's been a long time since I've done that.

After you've identified your top nurturing activities, post the list where you can see it easily. Each day, select at least one item and use it to nurture yourself.

TODAY

- Create your list of What I Love. Include at least twenty items.

- Mark any that you haven't done or appreciated in the past six months.

- Choose one thing from your list and use it today for nurturing or encouragement.

❧ DAY 34 ❧
Food replaces meaning

I once visited a national call center where rows of sales staff sat in low-walled cubicles. In between calls, many of the workers would flip up the mouthpiece on their headset, then eat from bags of food they kept in their top desk drawer. Handful after handful of chips, candy, cookies and trail mix went into the mouths of the staff members. Break times centered around the "potluck" table that held noodle casseroles and homemade cheesecake and brownies.

Sadly, nearly every person in this call center was overweight, many of them to a severe level of obesity. Yet many of them appeared to just push food into their mouths without even looking at what they were eating.

Meaning and connection

My guess is that for most of these people, the job wasn't very challenging or meaningful, so eating filled the empty places in their work life. If that sounds familiar, take a look at the amount of meaning in your own life right now.

Even if you can't change jobs or skip classes and events, you can work on building meaning in other areas. Perhaps it's time to join a book club or volunteer at a homeless shelter. Or pull out your recipe books and find meaning in creating healthy meals.

Do more self-care

Janice is a computer specialist who gets so engrossed in her work that she often sits for three to four hours without taking a break. Then her eyes feel tired, her back hurts, and she starts craving a candy bar to give her some quick energy.

Eventually, she realized her long periods without breaks were adding to her weight problem. So she found a way to set a timer on her computer to go off hourly. Now once an hour, she gets up, walks around, stretches a bit and drinks some water. Her new system has completely changed her patterns as well as helped her come home a lot less tired.

Identify some places during your day where you can slip in a little self-care activity. For example, set a timer for twenty minutes and make your meal or snack last that long. If nothing else, this will keep you from heading back to the buffet or potluck table for more helpings.

TODAY

- Write a list of things that currently give you meaning in your life.

- Decide where you can add more things or cultivate the ones you have.

- Do at least one activity that builds your sense of meaning. Record what you did.

❧ DAY 35 ❧
Need for renewal

When you continuously push through difficult days without taking a break, you can experience a weariness that doesn't let up. It's as though the core of your body, your inner spirit, is worn out. You still do your job, take care of your home and shuttle the kids to events. But there's no joy in your life. Maybe you have brief moments of fun and laughter, but an hour (or a day) later, the cloud is back. You've become life tired.

Self-nurturing activities such as taking a bath or listening to music can help. But sometimes, they aren't enough. You need a deeper level of healing, one that reaches your core and pulls it back up. You need renewal.

The renewal walk

Being life tired doesn't go away quickly. But you can take steps to renew your inner spirit. Start your renewal by taking a walk that is not designated as exercise. If you can't get outdoors, do your walk at a mall or even inside your office. Begin by focusing on your feet and noticing how they feel. Perhaps even take off your shoes and do this activity barefoot.

As you begin walking, let go of any thoughts, agendas and demands. Just keep noticing your feet. Pay attention to the way they move, how they feel and where they take you. Walk slowly and purposefully with openness to the world around you. Relax into your surroundings as you mentally and physically leave your problems behind.

After walking for a few minutes, move your focus upward and pay attention to your five senses: sight, hearing, smell, taste and touch. With each one, notice and experience things you might normally miss. Focus your eyes on something you haven't seen before. Listen for sounds you hadn't realized were there. Smell and taste something different and notice the sensations. Touch a specific object and observe its texture and character.

When you finish your walk, you may be surprised at how much better you feel. By narrowing your focus to nothing but your five senses, you shut out the rest of the world and give yourself a mini-nurturing break. With this simple act of connecting to your inner self, you can boost your energy and begin to find renewal.

TODAY

- Decide when you'll do a renewal walk. Allow plenty of time to focus on details.

- Record what you noticed or experienced with each of your five senses.

- Write notes about how your energy and your inner spirit felt after the renewal walk.

∾ DAY 36 ∾
My strengths

Megan is a graphic artist who works as a marketing director at a large company. She struggles with the demands of a challenging job as well as keeping balance in her home life with a husband and two young children. Over the past few years, a weight gain of almost 40 pounds has greatly affected her self-esteem.

To help her cope on days when she doesn't feel very competent or successful, I asked her to write a list of strengths based on what is almost true about herself. Creating her list wasn't easy because at that moment, she didn't see herself as attractive or competent.

Yet when she dug into her memories of how life had been in the past, she realized her skills and strengths were still there, even if she wasn't using them right now. Using my three suggested categories, Megan wrote the following list:

Physical attributes: Healthy, good weight, athletic, strong, attractive, pretty, appealing, sexy, active, energetic.
Skills and abilities: Intelligent, knowledgeable, quick learner, competent, organized, creative, detail oriented, good worker, quick thinker, decisive, confident, good parent.
Personality traits: Sensitive, intuitive, thoughtful, caring, kind, gentle, patient, loving, assertive, fun, enjoyable to be with.

Once she finished her list, Meagan was amazed at how much better she felt about herself and her capabilities. She realized her list reflected the way she was deep inside, even if she didn't always act that way.

Your list of strengths

Using the three categories above, create your own list of strengths. Include phrases such as good weight or physically fit even if right now your weight is up and you haven't exercised in a while.

Don't discount items on your list by saying, "I'm not really pretty or attractive or creative." Instead, hold tightly to the belief that you have these strengths, even during times when you don't feel them or do them. For example, even on a day when you yell at another driver or snap at a co-worker, you still are a kind and considerate person.

Over the next few weeks, read your list often. Any time you struggle with weak self-esteem or you doubt your abilities, use your list of strengths to renew your confidence and belief in yourself.

TODAY

- In your notebook, write "My strengths, even if I don't always believe them or do them."

- Using the categories of physical attributes, skills and abilities, and personality traits, create a list of your strengths.

- When you finish your list read it out loud. Write a note about how this feels.

❧ DAY 37 ❧
I'm not done yet

Some years ago, I visited one of my favorite college professors. This man gets some of the highest ratings possible from his students. He always seems to have a sparkle in his eyes. And when he talks about his classes, he practically jumps up and down. It's obvious that he loves his work and genuinely cares about his students.

But the amazing thing about this energetic, spirited professor is that at the time I visited with him, he was 76 years old! I was curious about his dedication to his work, so I asked him, "What keeps you teaching year after year? And when do you think you'll retire?"

"Oh my," he responded. "I don't plan on retiring any time soon. You see, I'm not done yet." I was surprised by this and said, "Really? What's left to do?" He laughed, then gave me his list:

- I'm not done helping students discover the treasure of education.
- I'm not done learning and studying in my field.
- I'm certainly not done caring for those who come to my classes.

I'm not done...

What an inspiration! His words got me thinking about lots of areas of my life that need pumped back up. And sometimes I need a way to create his level of enthusiasm. So now I have another self-talk phrase to boost my energy and commitment to my goals. For example, I'm not done ...

- Taking care of myself, physically as well as mentally and emotionally.
- Managing my weight, doing healthy eating and regular exercise.
- Caring about people in my work as well as in my personal life.

If I'm not done yet, I need to keep taking action. I've decided that at some point each day, I will remind myself, "Today, I'm staying on my eating plan, taking my walk, and doing some yoga stretches because…I'm not done yet!"

How about you? What are some areas where you aren't done yet? Of course, some things are ongoing, such as raising children, getting a college degree or remodeling your kitchen. But in terms of your weight-loss and exercise goals, think about areas where you would truly say you aren't done yet. Start building your list, then figure out the action steps it will take to continue making progress on those areas.

TODAY

- Identify at least three things or life areas you aren't done with yet.

- Decide on steps you can take today on each of these items.

- With each of those actions, record that you've completed them.

✨ DAY 38 ✨
Emotional cold

Have you been struggling with life lately? Maybe feeling a bit down? I'm wondering if you might have an emotional cold. With this type of cold, you feel a little moody, discouraged and slightly depressed. You aren't dealing with deep issues that need counseling or medication. You just feel an emotional letdown or a sense of emptiness.

An emotional cold can be brought on by any number of stressful things. Sometimes it's a struggling relationship, a job layoff or just being overwhelmed or sick of life at the moment.

In some cases, work demands or an ill parent can wear you out. Often you'll recognize your emotional cold by the way you keep reaching for cookies or chips when you thought you'd conquered those foods.

Here are three steps to help you recover from an emotional cold:

1. Admit it's a real cold

Give up the fake happy face and admit that you're feeling down. With an emotional cold, you can't just talk yourself out of it, ignore it or shake it off. You may just have to snuggle under an emotional blanket for a few days and give yourself time to get better.

2. Don't blame yourself

Even if you realize it's related to stress or not taking time for yourself, getting an emotional cold is not your fault. It just shows up, often as a way to remind you to slow down and take better care of yourself.

If you eat sweets or junk food in your efforts to cope with your cold, don't conclude that you're weak or a failure. You probably just needed some relief from the symptoms while you waited for life to heal you.

3. Nurture yourself until you feel better

Do lots of self-care activities while you allow yourself time to recover. Take some emotional time off. Call in sick (because you have a "bad cold") or ask your family to help out more for a few days because of your "illness." Once you've recovered and you're feeling better, renew your determination for healthy eating and exercise.

Everyone gets an emotional cold now and then. If you learn to recognize the symptoms and start treating it right away, you'll perk back up and recover a lot faster.

TODAY

- Create a first-aid kit for the next time you get an emotional cold.

- Write a list of things you can do to help you recover when one hits.

- Do one of the things on your list today. It might help prevent you from getting an emotional cold.

∽ DAY 39 ∾
See your value

Vicki blamed herself for her weight gain. At her highest weight of 320 pounds, she was so miserable she could barely stand to look at herself in the mirror. Worst of all, she kept telling herself she was a failure and that she wasn't ever going to be able to change.

When Vicki got on a plane to visit her family, she maneuvered herself into the seat by the window and tried to take up as little room as possible. But minutes later, she heard a loud male voice announce to the flight attendant, "I'm sorry, but you'll have to reassign me to another seat. This lady is taking up so much room, I couldn't possibly fit comfortably in the row with her."

This humiliation only added to the negative phrases Vicki was already telling herself. But an hour into the flight, Vicki felt a hand on her shoulder. When she raised her head, she looked into the kind face of a flight attendant who said, "I apologize for that insensitive man. Don't let him ruin your day! You are a valuable person and don't ever tell yourself that you aren't!"

Vicki was stunned. No one had ever said she was a valuable person! She also realized that everything she'd been telling herself was the exact opposite. At that moment, Vicki straightened her shoulders and made a decision. She was going to start living like a valuable person.

Changing your self-talk

During the remainder of the flight, Vicki began telling herself, "You are a beautiful woman. You are strong and capable. You are valuable to the world." And by the end of the flight, she started believing her own words.

She also vowed she would never face a situation like that again. After Vicki returned home, she joined a new weight-loss program and lost 165 pounds. In addition to maintaining a healthy weight, Vicki now mentors other women and helps them achieve weight-loss success, partly by changing their self-talk.

You are valuable!

The words you say to yourself can affect nearly everything you do. Starting today, change the negative words you say to yourself. Instead of saying "I can't do anything right," hold your head up high and tell yourself, "I'm important, I'm valuable, and I count in this world."

TODAY

- Create two positive statements to use for your self-talk.

- Write them on a card or piece of paper, then post them where you can read them often.

- Live as if these statements are true, then record your response.

ᔏ DAY 40 ᔐ
Believe in yourself

Imagine you're walking through a forest when you spot a large piece of wood nearly hidden in a pile of leaves. As you study the layers of moss and caked-on dirt, you can't see any beauty in this scrap of wood and you question whether it has any value. But something compels you to pick it up and carry it home. In your workshop, you carefully scrape off the dirt, then begin sanding and polishing the wood. To your astonishment, you uncover a deep grain filled with rich, beautiful colors.

As you continue restoring the wood, you start planning how you could use it for some special purpose. Your excitement builds as you envision creating a unique picture frame or a graceful table leg. There's no doubt in your mind this piece of wood has great value.

You are this piece of wood. Even when painful layers such as your weight or other burdens cover your beauty, the real you never leaves. Beneath your discouragement and low self-esteem, you are still you, as strong and vibrant as ever.

Restore your spirit

It's so easy to let events or situations ruin your confidence. Even when you've worked hard on building your self-esteem, a simple negative comment can destroy your inner spirit and send you running toward the refrigerator.

And it works, because food makes you feel good! When something devastates your confidence or your self-trust, eating soothes the pain and gives you courage to face the world again.

Of course, at the same time, overeating actually harms your self-esteem by making you feel disgusted and frustrated. So you grab more food to appease your negative feelings. And that just makes you feel even worse!

Regardless of your current life situation, you can still find your inner spirit and rebuild your self-esteem. And it won't take years to accomplish. By making a few simple changes in your self-talk and your internal beliefs, you can improve your self-esteem almost immediately.

Think back to the earlier example of the piece of wood. You may have to scrape off a few old beliefs and habits, but you can build self-esteem that remains strong, no matter what happens in your life. Soon, your renewed self-image will add power to your efforts for managing your weight.

TODAY

- Write the words "I am valuable" in your notebook.

- Consider ways you can restore your belief in your own value. Describe them.

- Do at least one action today that will demonstrate your sense of value and self-worth. Record what you did.

DAYS 31–40 COMPLETED!

You've come this far in your 100 days...

Don't stop now. If you're struggling to stick with it, push yourself to finish *one more day*. You'll immediately be another day closer to achieving your weight-loss goals.

Just do one more day!

❧ DAYS 41–50 ❧

SEPARATE EMOTIONS AND FOOD

✎ DAY 41 ✎
Food and feelings

Karen is a highly successful businesswoman who has built a consulting company based on her ability to resolve conflicts and devise management solutions. But in her own life, though, she admits that food becomes her solace, giving her the comfort and validation that's often missing in her workdays. Karen told me, "I don't eat food, I use food."

It happens so easily. At some point in life, food becomes your friend. Unfortunately, this friend encourages you to bury your uncomfortable feelings and simply eat more to keep them stuffed away. This friend also seduces you into believing your crummy life actually isn't so bad as long as you have chocolate or potato chips.

At times, you depend on this friend for all of your enjoyment in life. But at the same time you're comforting or entertaining yourself with food, you secretly know this friend is ruining your life.

Food works

Emotional eating or using food as a friend happens to all of us at times. This type of eating serves a purpose, usually appeasing emotional needs or thought patterns. It also fixes things such as low self-esteem or feeling like a failure as well as emotions ranging from anger to despair.

Emotional eating can be obvious, like searching the cupboards when you are bored or lonely. But sometimes the struggles are more hidden, such as eating to bury painful emotions or avoid reality.

Jane told me, "For years I put up with a bad marriage that didn't have any fun, excitement or nurturing. I didn't want to face how bad things were, and I didn't have the courage to leave. So I ate all day long and pretended everything was fine."

Changing these patterns won't come easily. You may like the way food comforts and nurtures you. Instant relief appeals more than facing emotional needs and working on your personal growth. In many cases, eating is easier than thinking.

But I encourage you to keep learning how to identify and express your emotions rather than shoving them away with food. As you develop new coping skills, you'll be able to change your friendship with food into a healthy relationship.

TODAY

- List three of the most common times or situations where you do emotional eating.

- For each one, add details including what might be going on or causing you to eat.

- Then for each one, write a plan for how you can take care of the real issue instead of reaching for food. Watch for times to use this today.

❧ DAY 42 ❧
Food and fun

For some people, food provides an escape from the drudgery of life. Jerry told me, "I work in a dead-end job, my marriage is awful, and my kids are always in trouble. We constantly struggle with money, barely covering our bills each month. Most days, food is the only thing I have to look forward to. It's all I've got."

Food entertains us with no strings attached. If you can't find something you like on TV, you can raid the refrigerator until the programs change. On rainy afternoons or long weekends with no plans, food helps fill the empty time. In fact, Jerry admitted, "Without food, I'd have no fun at all!"

When your life is stressful or unhappy, food makes the world more bearable. Later, when the painful realities of your life return, you simply eat again. It seems quicker and easier than trying to invent new ways to entertain yourself or to cope with life challenges.

Food provides transitions

Have you noticed how food also provides a convenient way to move from one event or time of day to another? Doughnuts start a meeting. Dessert ends a meal. Ice cream signifies bedtime. Even your afternoon snack indicates you are home from work and ready to start your evening.

After a stressful workday, Kevin decided to stop at a fast-food restaurant on the way home. The next day, he did it again. Before he knew it, he'd slipped into the habit of going through the drive-up lane every day after work. After a year of transition snacks of french fries and milkshakes, Kevin had gained more than fifty pounds.

To break this pattern, Kevin decided to shake up his routine. He drove home from work on a different street and turned into his driveway from the opposite direction. Rather than entering his house through the garage, he switched to the front door, then immediately walked upstairs instead of toward the kitchen.

In your own life, you may need to invent new ways to manage transitions in your day. You can mark being off work by drinking hot tea or a diet soda. Change your bedtime routine to include relaxing music or stretching exercises instead of a bowl of ice cream.

TODAY

- Identify places or times when food provides your main source of fun or entertainment.

- Make a list of creative, non-food ways to have fun. Do one of them today.

- For situations where food provides a transition, invent ways to shake up your routine and follow a healthier pattern.

✤ DAY 43 ✤
Food memories

Have you ever heard an old song on the radio and suddenly remembered a person or an event you hadn't thought about in years? Maybe it reminded you of your first love or a great concert or a party. Just like that familiar old song, your favorite foods can also be connected to situations from your past.

Foods often become embedded in your memory, not just because of how they taste, but because of the feelings you originally had around them. Each time you associate a particular food with an event or an experience, you create a link that continues to exist even years later.

For example, suppose you are at a baseball game and you get an overwhelming desire for a hot dog. Is it because you love the taste of hot dogs? Or is it because you love the feelings stirred by memories of fun times when you attended ball games as a child?

We tend to miss the happiness and comfort of good times in our past. By eating a memory-associated food, we attempt to recapture those wonderful old feelings. But since we can't return to those experiences, food becomes as close as we get.

Food connections

See if you can remember times in your childhood when you ate some of your favorite foods. Recall where you were and the people you were with at those times. Here are some examples that might help you pull up your own food memories.

94

- Ice cream cones: Saturday night. We made a special trip into town and bought ice cream to celebrate the end of a week.
- Pink cotton candy: Annual trip to the circus. It was one of the few times Dad and I went to an event by ourselves.
- Three-layer chocolate cake: My birthday. I got to pick out the cake. It was a time when I felt noticed and valued.

By tracing back to your earliest recollections of eating a food, you can identify the needs that were met at that time. When you crave that food now, you are probably experiencing some of the same needs as in your food memory.

TODAY

- List several favorite foods that often cause you problems or tempt you to overeat.

- Recall events or places where you have eaten these foods, especially as a child. Describe the scenes, including the people you were with.

- Identify one or two emotions that seem the strongest in each scene. Record your insights including times when that food connects to emotions now.

❧ DAY 44 ❧
Food tracing

I really like cookies. But I could never figure out why they tempted me so much at certain times. When I did a food tracing, I was amazed to learn that my love of cookies was connected to childhood memories of feeling warm, safe and secure. I've learned that when I start craving cookies, I'm usually feeling insecure or emotionally unsafe somewhere in my life.

Do you have specific foods that you crave at odd times? Like my cookies, tracing your memories back to your earliest recollection of eating a food will often identify the exact emotional needs that were met at that time.

How to do a food tracing

Pick a favorite food that often causes you problems or tempts you to overeat. Close your eyes and mentally track backward to events or places where you have eaten this food. You might remember celebrations, specific friends, or perhaps lonely or difficult periods in your life.

Think back to your childhood and focus on your earliest memories of eating this food. Picture the scene in detail. Where are you? Who else is present? What are you feeling as you are eating this food? Are you warm, comforted, happy, peaceful, safe, nurtured? Are you escaping from negative emotions such as anger or fear? Is this food memory associated with a time of grief or sadness?

Perhaps you recall a time when your family was happier or more peaceful than usual. Identify one or two emotions that seem the strongest in this picture. Open your eyes and record your insights.

Connect to today

Now think of your present struggles with this food. When you crave it most, are you experiencing some of the same needs as you were in your food-tracing memory? When emotional needs arise, these vague food memories may actually drive you to seek the relief you found in the past.

You may be surprised at what pops to mind when you look for the memories that hook you with your favorite food. Food tracing will often reveal thoughts of better days when your needs for comfort, nurturing and happiness were met.

TODAY

- Choose a favorite food and write down times when you seem to crave it a lot.

- Close your eyes and mentally track backward to your earliest memories of eating this food. Describe the scene, then add the emotions you were feeling at that time.

- Connect those emotions or needs to present times when you crave this food. Record your insights as well as some non-food ways to take care of these needs.

❧ DAY 45 ❧
Safe places

Once you outgrew your pacifier as a child, you probably looked for something else to make you feel safe and content. Maybe you slept with a tattered blanket or a scruffy stuffed animal in your bed. But where are the teddy bears in your life today? Even though you've outgrown your toys, sometimes you still need an emotional security blanket.

For many of us, food makes us feel comforted as well as safe. But the feelings don't last long, and soon we look for more food to fill the anxiety or emptiness inside. One of the most powerful ways to change this pattern is to identify a safe place where you can give yourself a break from the stresses of life.

Create a safe place

In your home or work setting, look for a room or even a corner that you can turn into a safe place. Fill this area with favorite objects that make you feel secure and comfortable. Personalize your safe place by adding posters, candles or stuffed animals. Consider adding a plant or a colorful silk arrangement to brighten your mood.

Once you create your safe place, go there often. Read, listen to music or simply allow yourself to feel calm and secure. Even a few minutes can be long enough to renew your spirit. Over time, you'll discover amazing things in your safe place and none of them will require food.

Safety on the run

You can create emotional safety anywhere. For example, you might keep a variety of music options in your car to ease tension while you are driving. Carry a favorite coffee cup to meetings. It will give you something familiar to hold on to, especially during tense discussions.

Watch for specific places you can use as an oasis or a safe retreat. A nearby park, your car, even a neighborhood coffee shop can all be turned into safe places to temporarily hide or regroup when you need to.

Whenever you're going through a major change in life, emotional safety is especially important. Any time you start a new job or move to a different home, don't wait for months to "fix things up." Take immediate steps to make yourself feel comfortable and emotionally safe, even in a brand-new setting.

TODAY

- Write a plan for creating a safe place.

- Set up and personalize the area. Describe what's in your safe place and how it looks.

- Spend at least ten minutes in your safe place today. Write about what you did and how it felt.

∾ DAY 46 ∾
Disappointment

It all started when the dentist announced I had a cracked filling that needed to be replaced with a crown. What I thought was going to cost a few hundred dollars suddenly jumped to an estimate of over one thousand!

From there, things kept adding up until I became a total grouch. I yelled nasty things at my husband and threw stuffed toys at my dog. (I was tired of tripping over them.)

I could see it coming. I was only inches away from reaching for a carton of my favorite ice cream. But before giving in to my food cravings, I decided to remind myself about other ways to cope with disappointment.

When life lets you down

You probably understand disappointment all too well. From your first broken toy to the partner or the job that got away, you certainly recognize the ache of losing something important to you.

Disappointment happens to us all the time. With the small ones, we treat them as simply being minor issues in our day. Other times, coping with disappointment isn't so easy. When a major loss shatters your life dreams, bouncing back takes a lot more effort. And unless you are able to do some healing and nurturing, food will become an easy and appealing solution.

Find the "trade-offs"

Whenever you feel disappointed because something didn't go the way you wanted, look for the trade-off you got instead. Maybe you learned or experienced something new. Perhaps a different opportunity or item showed up instead of the one you wanted so badly.

Although a trade-off doesn't replace what you originally wanted, sometimes it presents an even better solution. For example, if you are disappointed about not getting a new job, your trade-off might be having less stress and a shorter commute. When you can't get tickets to a sold-out concert, you might download the music so you can hear your favorite songs every day.

Trade-offs don't mean you aren't disappointed. You still need to acknowledge your feelings and your sense of loss. But remind yourself that food won't magically make the loss go away. Then instead of letting a disappointment pull you into despair, search for the trade-offs and give yourself a new perspective.

TODAY

- Write down a recent disappointment. It can be a small one or a larger, life disappointment.

- Record your initial response, including whether it made you want to eat something.

- Look for a "trade-off" or what you got instead. Describe this in detail.

❦ DAY 47 ❧
Food replaces love

Every year in May, we celebrate Mother's Day here in the United States. For me, it's always a difficult holiday.

As many of you know, I was not able to have children. I was born with a defective uterus that couldn't support a full-term pregnancy. Three different times, I carried a pregnancy for six months before going into premature labor. Two of my baby girls were stillborn. The third one lived for eleven hours before leaving this earth.

For many years, I used food to help me deal with my grief. Whenever I felt sad about my babies, I would eat a lot and try to avoid thinking. My weight-loss efforts never lasted because I always ended up trying to eat away the painful memories of losing my babies.

Many of you have similar issues with the Mother's Day holiday. Perhaps your own mother has died or you've lost a child. Maybe you had family problems that created a chasm between you and your mother.

So how do you cope with these empty life places without filling them with food? In my own life, I had to learn how to stop burying my emotions and allow myself to feel. I also had to figure out that there isn't enough food in the world to fix my empty heart.

Switching the pattern

Connie always felt let down by her children on Mother's Day. Usually she spent much of the day eating to deal with her anger and frustration. One year she decided to rename the holiday, "Glad I'm your mother day."

Now instead of hoping for cards and phone calls, she reaches out to each of her children and offers encouragement and support for whatever goals they are working on. She ends by thanking them for being her children. This simple change completely stopped her Mother's Day overeating and left her feeling blessed and thankful.

With holidays or birthdays, it doesn't matter how strongly you believe someone should call, visit or be nice to you. Instead of waiting for someone to show you love, try turning the tables and giving it out. Remember that you hold the power for your own nurturing and you don't have to use food to replace love.

TODAY

- Identify a holiday, birthday or event where you wait for someone to care about you.

- Plan ways you can show extra love and attention to others during this time.

- Notice how it changes your desire to eat in order to cope. Record your response.

❧ DAY 48 ❧
Stress is not life

When Sherry started her current job, she liked being out of the house and helping with the family bills. Then she was promoted to a manager position that turned out to be extremely difficult. Besides her constant struggle with feeling tired and overwhelmed, she missed the days when she didn't feel so stressed.

Sherry's constant stress, both at work and at home, kept sending her to the doughnut box or bag of potato chips. Food not only calmed her back down, it also gave her a bit of respite and enjoyment in her overwhelming life.

Maybe eating will help...

When people list their reasons for emotional eating, stress usually ranks at the top. We use food to get through everything from divorce and family illness to struggles with jobs and parenting. Even if you've maintained your weight for a long time, a stressful event can push you instantly back into old patterns of eating for relief.

To stop this type of emotional eating, you either have to cope with stress differently or change the way you view it. I think it's time to go back to labeling stress as being a piece of your day, not a way of life.

The broken leg approach

Even though I'd never wish this on anyone, think about what would happen if you broke your leg. When you picture recovering from your injury, you will soon realize you aren't as indispensable as you thought.

Imagine all the places you'd suddenly have to make changes or eliminate responsibilities. Now pick out a few of those demands and, using the broken leg approach, make changes in them right now. Take control by deciding which activities are critical to keep and which ones you can let go.

You might even explain to your family or your boss that recent events require you to take a break from some of your demands. Ask for help in deciding which things can wait a few weeks or even be totally eliminated. You may be surprised at how much your stress decreases when you have a "broken leg."

When you feel stressed, look specifically at what's causing the pressure. Then make changes wherever possible to protect yourself from too many demands.

TODAY

- Identify one area in life that tempts you to eat in response to stress.

- Describe how you will cope with this area differently due to your "broken leg."

- Record ways your new plan helped you manage your stress without eating.

∽ DAY 49 ∼
Laugh away stress

Some years ago, I invited several families to help celebrate my husband's birthday. We had a full house, with kids ranging from 6 to 16 years old. We requested that everyone spend one hour during this visit without cell phones and video games.

I worried the kids might get bored without their technology and not enjoy the evening. But you'll be amazed at what they did—they laughed! At everything! They made up jokes, they invented pretend people and they laughed at each other's silliness.

During this time, the adults chatted around the dining room table. We had warm and caring conversation, but guess what? We didn't laugh. Sure, we giggled a few times, but never the hilarious, belly-clutching laughter of the kids.

Stress takes away fun

Brian described the stress of working at a high-pressure technology firm. He said, "My life is nothing but demands and pressure. I miss having fun, and I want to go back to the days when I could play and laugh and roll in the grass!"

I think laughter could be a great cure for stress-related eating. But when your life is filled with burdens and worries, how do you get back to feeling light-hearted? Maybe you just need to give yourself a chance to laugh and play the way you used to.

Have a play date

Set up a play date for yourself, just like parents do for their children. Your play date can be done alone or with other people. Think about what would make you laugh, then plan something that will be fun and entertaining.

If you love movies, designate going to a movie as your play date. Select which one you'll see, then check where it's playing and what time it starts. Give yourself permission to have fun on your play date, even if you see a bad movie.

Other play dates might involve going dancing, playing board games, listening to live bands or meeting a friend for tea. Set your play dates around activities that give you a break from the pressures in your life. Soon you'll discover that laughter and fun will relieve stress much better than a carton of ice cream.

TODAY

- Create a plan for a play date for yourself, either alone or with another person.

- Set a day and time for your play date and write down what you will do.

- Afterward, describe your play date and how it helped you relax, laugh and have fun.

✎ DAY 50 ✎
Empty bucket

Picture a large container such as a water bucket. Inside this bucket, you have a constantly shifting level of positive emotional energy. When you are feeling healthy and balanced in your life, your bucket level will be at least half-full. Ideally, you start each day this way.

But just like physical energy, you have a limited amount of emotional energy. As you go through your day, demands from people, job or family stress, even the weather can take a toll on it. At the same time, positive things increase the level in your bucket. Kindness, affirmations, self-care and nurturing can all help restore the level.

If you have lots of positive things in your life, your emotional energy climbs and life feels good. But during times when you have a lot of negatives or drainers, your emotional energy drops below the minimal level. By the end of the day, you are exhausted emotionally as well as physically.

If you don't refill the bucket at intervals, you can reach a point where it's empty day after day. Unfortunately, this often leads to reaching for food to try to fill that empty space. In your efforts to stop running on empty, food becomes an easy solution.

Emotional energy is essential to living in a healthy and balanced way. If you ignore your empty bucket too long, you can struggle with depression, low self-esteem and lost motivation.

Filling your emotional bucket

While food might help you feel better for a while, it doesn't give you the kind of energy you need in your emotional bucket. Instead, think about what fuels you and helps you feel more positive. Maybe it's time to read a book or have a quiet cup of coffee. Put on your headphones and let the music build your spirits.

Look for positive people who are energy builders instead of drainers. Draw on things that nurture you or increase your meaning in life. Create a list of things that work and pull it out whenever your bucket level feels low.

By taking care of your emotional bucket at intervals, you'll prevent it from getting so low you feel drained and empty. Each day, plan a few things that will fill your level of emotional energy back up, even just a little.

TODAY

- Write a list of things that drain your emotional energy.

- Write a second list of things that build your emotional energy back up.

- Evaluate the current level of your emotional bucket and plan ways to improve it daily.

DAYS 41–50 COMPLETED!

You've come this far in your 100 days...

Don't stop now. If you're struggling to stick with it, push yourself to finish *one more day*. You'll immediately be another day closer to achieving your weight-loss goals.

Just do one more day!

❧ DAYS 51–60 ❧

FIX THE REAL NEEDS

❧ DAY 51 ❧
Emotional needs

After her divorce, Kaye struggled a lot with emotional eating. She said, "I miss so many things I used to have in my life. I wish I had time to sit outside under a tree and read a good book. I miss being held, making special dinners, being appreciated or having a slow day without all my stress.

"I need a lot of things, but since I can't seem to get them, I reach for food instead. A bag of chips or cookies replaces the happy home I wish I had. Snacks in my work drawer fill in for the compliments I'm not getting. The bowl of ice cream late at night takes the place of arms around me."

What do I need?
We all have needs in our lives. But to deal with them in ways that don't involve food, you need to become skilled at knowing what you are trying to fix. Here's a great method for identifying your emotional needs.

At the top of a blank piece of paper, write the question, "What do I need?" Using one or two words or short phrases, begin making a list of things you are lacking or missing in your life. Each time you record a need, ask the question again, saying, "What else do I need?"

Consider needs related to your weight, self-esteem, stress, job and relationships. Include small needs such as money or rest, as well as complex ones such as a new job or a different life partner.

Keep answering the "What do I need" question until you have exhausted your thoughts and can't come up with any more answers.

Once you finish, read through the needs you identified. Most likely, your initial list will include things such as the desire for nurturing, less stress or more money. But you may also find words such as safety, affirmation, intimacy or even escape.

As you know from figuring out what you feel, labeling gives you power. So while identifying what you need won't always stop you from emotional eating, at least it will help you see the connection of how food takes care of you.

TODAY

- Write the words, "What do I need?" Then make a list of your needs. Keep asking the question, "What else do I need?" until you have at least ten things.

- Put a check mark or star by the ones that are most important right now.

- Choose one thing from your list and do something today that will help take care of that need.

ೲ DAY 52 ಌ
The food fix

G ary is a psychologist with a busy private practice. He told me, "I don't know how my life got so out of hand. My days fly by but I never get caught up with all my tasks. I feel like I'm missing a lot of things, and I suspect I'm using food to replace them."

Here's Gary's list of needs:

Time—I wish I wasn't always behind and trying to get
  caught up.
Closeness—more intimacy with my wife, feeling closer to
  my kids.
Connection—time with people who are authentic,
  encouraging and not so demanding.
Fun—more enjoyment of life, not so burdened by all my
  required activities.
Hope—see the potential for life to get better instead of
  being so pessimistic about it.
Feel settled—instead of restless and constantly searching
  for meaning.

As he reviewed his list, Gary began to understand what food was doing for him. It was taking the place of everything he yearned for in life but didn't have.

Security and emotional safety

Sometimes you won't recognize that emotional needs are sending you toward food. For example, during times when you feel anxious or afraid, eating provides stamina. When life challenges affect your confidence, eating boosts your courage.

Perhaps you eat a snack before presenting your big project at work. Or you grab a few cookies before calling your ex-husband about the child-support payments. As long as you have food, you feel strong enough to deal with difficult issues.

If you feel nervous or uncomfortable at a party, you can just hide your feelings behind a plate of snacks. When uneasiness creeps back in, you can simply eat more. Food becomes the security blanket that gets you through the evening.

No quick fix

As you work on identifying your needs, don't get stuck by saying, "I can't do anything about that!" Right now, your task is to figure out exactly what is contributing to your emotional eating. You won't be able to fix all of these needs right away, but knowing what they are will help you recognize where to start making changes.

TODAY

- Look back at the list of needs you made yesterday. Now add a list of deeper needs such as better self-esteem or more motivation.

- For each of these deeper needs, note the times when you use food to fix them.

- Choose one of those needs and create an action plan for taking care of it without food.

❧ DAY 53 ❧
Taking care of needs

How do you change your eating patterns when your needs are so great and food is so easy? When you can't find a minute to yourself during the day, where do you start?

As much as you wish someone else would fix your life, ultimately you have to do it yourself. Even if you believe that your family or boss or lover should do more for you, other people can never fill all the gaps in your life.

It's up to you to figure out how to get your needs met. This may require moving yourself up on your priority list, ahead of your aging mother or your demanding boss.

Fixing your needs

Take out the list of needs you created over the past two days. You may want to add a few more items for today. For example, if you are going to a party or visiting your mother, consider the question, "What do I need during this event or activity?"

Now add a column to the other side of your paper and write, "How could I get it?" Then for each item on your list, identify what it would take to get that specific need met, even partially, and record your answers.

Consider every possible solution that might appease your emotional needs, at least long enough to keep you out of the refrigerator. With deeper needs, identify one or two small steps that will move you toward success.

Once you create solutions that would meet your needs, make them happen. Take a walk, close your office door, hug your child. Often one simple action can redirect how you manage your entire day. What seemed so overwhelming that you had pushed it away with food suddenly becomes more bearable.

Remember Kaye, who was struggling after her divorce? After writing her list of needs, she looked at all the ways she could get those needs met in spite of her sadness about her marriage.

Within a week, she felt more in charge of her life. She said, "Doing those simple things took away a lot of the food cravings I'd been fighting for so long. Instead of eating to make my life go away, I discovered I had the power to heal my own pain."

TODAY

- When you wake up each morning, ask yourself "What do I need today?" Record several things.

- For each item, write an answer to the question, "How can I get it?"

- Choose one need, then make an action plan for working on it today.

∽ DAY 54 ∾
Please comfort me

Don knew that food often filled in for what was missing in his life. He told me, "On Friday night, I had planned to go to a movie, but when I got to the theater, the show was sold out. So I stopped at the video store on the way home and rented a movie instead. It turned out to be horrible—not the slightest bit entertaining or enjoyable. But the evening wasn't a total loss. I had my pint of butter pecan ice cream, so that became my fun."

Don was also afraid that if he couldn't use food for comfort, he wouldn't be able to cope. He said, "For me, food helps me survive. Overeating is like pushing the mute button on my life. But I keep doing it, because if I stop, life feels too awful to deal with."

The comfort of food

When I was a child, I remember falling and skinning my knee, then having my mom give me a cookie and say, "Here you go. Now you'll feel better." And my skinned knee magically stopped hurting.

As an adult, I still find that a few cookies can take away emotional pain in my life. You may have a similar pattern. Whenever you face a difficult situation, you think, "If I eat something, maybe I'll feel better." Besides, it feels really cozy to curl up under a blanket with a bowl of ice cream or a couple of brownies.

For many people, food takes care of all types of needs. It even provides an anchor when you move or get a new job.

As you scramble to adjust to new surroundings, you realize that food didn't change. Once you locate a familiar fast-food restaurant, you suddenly feel better. You can travel, start a new job or move far away and food will still be there!

Even if you've been an emotional eater for years, you aren't stuck with these negative patterns. Start by realizing the key to managing your weight begins with healing your heart, not filling your spoon. As you discover new ways to cope with your emotional needs, you'll move toward a sense of peace with food—a feeling you may have forgotten existed.

TODAY

- Recall a recent time when food helped you feel comforted or secure. Describe it.

- Come up with at least two or three things you could have done instead of eating.

- Write a plan about how you'll use one of those items the next time you need comfort.

∽ DAY 55 ∾
Food as a reward

Every day you work hard at your job. You meticulously clean your house. You take good care of your children. After these efforts, you feel like you deserve a reward but no one gives you one. Sometimes you get the opposite such as criticism or verbal abuse. So you reward yourself—by eating.

Professionals such as teachers and nurses tell me they rarely get any positive feedback or appreciation. In their work, they are expected to be patient, kind and giving to everyone else. When they don't receive anything in return, food can easily become the reward for their efforts.

In our busy, chaotic lives, we sometimes want a break from all of our demands and responsibilities. When we eat, we tell our hectic thoughts, "Here's a small reward. It will help you get through the rest of your day."

As a psychotherapist, Carla spent long days doing intense counseling sessions with her clients. In addition to keeping up on paperwork and attending committee meetings, she supervised new therapists on staff.

One afternoon, as she crammed down a candy bar, Carla noticed how calm she felt. She said, "For a few seconds, my brain focused on my mouth instead of the other thoughts flying through my head. It felt like I was rewarded for my work in the middle of my crazy day."

Planning a reward
Perhaps you've even set up your own reward system. By promising you can eat afterwards, you get motivated

to clean up the yard or study for an exam. You may even convince yourself you deserve food because of what you've accomplished or the efforts you've made.

But rewarding yourself with food results in a hollow victory. In reality, you would much rather be noticed by the people you worked so hard to please. If only your boss would commend your work or your spouse would express appreciation, maybe you wouldn't feel compelled to reach for a food reward.

It's time to come up with a non-food way to get rewards in your life. For example, write your own praise letter and tell yourself the words you need to hear. It's not the same as a big chocolate-chip cookie, but the kind words will give you a nice reward without making you gain weight.

TODAY

- Create a list of non-food rewards. At least once today, reward yourself with something from your list.

- Write a praise letter for something you've done. Email or send it to yourself.

- Give rewards such as hugs, cards or appreciation to others. Record your actions.

❧ DAY 56 ❧
I'm so bored

When there's nothing on TV and no one to talk to, you may end up wandering around the house and decide you're bored. Unfortunately, when you feel bored, you get something to eat. But here's an interesting thought. In reality, you may not be bored at all. Instead, you might be yearning for a new relationship or to feel challenged.

Maybe you wish you had something to do that involves connection with people or has meaning attached to it. You'd prefer to go to the latest movie with another person, then heatedly discuss the plot while drinking cappuccinos. You'd like to discover a musician whose interpretation of a classical piece moves you to tears.

Sometimes, you want memory makers that will stick with you later. You want to remember a special event and feel the enjoyment again the next day. In reality, you aren't really bored. Instead, you are seeking things that will add meaning and connection to your life.

Instead of labeling this as boredom, experiment with reviving interests from your past or learning some new skills. Once you pull them back out, you might remember how much you enjoyed crafts such as needlepoint and embroidery. Perhaps this is a time to start gardening or woodworking.

Consider experimenting with creative writing such as poetry or short stories. Even recording your thoughts in a journal can add meaning by helping you sort your ideas and feelings.

Wanting a challenge

Even when you have lots to do and you have plenty of friends or people to relate to, you might still feel empty and unfulfilled. You'd love to enjoy a deeper level of excitement, newness or personal growth. What you want is a challenge.

Instead of searching the cupboards, consider developing new skills in an area that interests you. Perhaps you could study astronomy or participate in an archeological dig. Maybe you could challenge yourself each day to do small deeds of kindness that will make a difference in someone's life. Volunteer at a school and tutor someone in reading or math.

Any time you are feeling bored, take a few minutes to determine what's prompting your thoughts. Then use solutions that match your specific needs instead of eating because you are bored.

TODAY

- Create a challenge list to use next time you feel bored. Include things that will give you meaning or deepen your knowledge and skills.

- Do at least one of the things on your list today.

- Record how that worked and whether it helped you avoid food temptations.

❧ DAY 57 ❧
People make me eat

Some years ago, I routinely met a good friend at a coffee shop where we would catch up on the events in our lives. My friend would usually debate whether or not to order a doughnut. Because I wanted to feel close to her, I would give in and say, "If you want a doughnut, I'll have one too."

After a while, I realized that my desire to connect was ruining my diet plan. So I changed my approach and simply said, "Go ahead and have one if you like. I'm not that hungry today, so I'll just have coffee."

When we want to connect with people, food becomes the string that pulls us together. Sometimes your efforts to connect don't even work. After a disappointing date or a dull party, you may still yearn to feel close to people. Heading to the refrigerator might seem like a good solution, but food can't make up for the absence of good companionship or meaningful conversation.

It's not my fault

Most of us don't like conflict, so when someone tells us to eat, we do it. We get caught up in pleasing other people, even when that harms our own goals. Families often have unspoken expectations around food. At family gatherings, people may expect you to stuff yourself with pasta or ice cream because "this is how we always eat."

My clients will often defend themselves by saying, "What was I supposed to do? They begged me to join them and I didn't want to hurt their feelings." Of course, whenever you eat to avoid hurting people's feelings, you hurt yourself instead.

When you eat because it's expected, you meet someone else's need for power. Barbara said, "For years, I endured the snide comments my husband's relatives made whenever I tried to lose weight. Usually, I'd just give in and take second helpings and eat dessert along with everyone else.

"One day it hit me that by eating to please my in-laws, I was sacrificing my weight-loss goals to keep peace in the family. So I made a decision that I would take care of my own needs instead of eating to please them. Eventually they stopped pushing me to overeat."

TODAY

- Identify situations where you eat to please someone or because it's expected.

- Write a statement that describes how you will avoid giving away your power by eating to please others.

- Create a plan for managing the situations where you eat to please someone. Put it in place today.

๑ DAY 58 ๛

Grieve your progress

When my husband retired a few years ago, we moved to another state to be closer to family. It was a good move, but instead of feeling excited and happy, I had moments when I felt incredibly sad.

I missed my window above the sink and my huge garden with lots of flowers. I also missed my friends, my church and my favorite restaurants. And I learned that even the best changes in life can leave you feeling sad and disappointed. I call this grieving your progress.

Leaving the past behind

A few weeks before we moved, my husband and I sat in our cozy loft one last time and toasted our home and the years we'd lived there. We talked about many wonderful times, but we also recalled a lot of sad moments such as the job interviews that never went anywhere, the deaths of our parents and my challenge of having breast cancer.

As we talked about our plans for moving to the new house, we felt excited, but also very sad. And we grieved our progress.

Recognize what you're leaving

Every time you get on the scale, you mark your progress. But in spite of strong goals and a desire to lose weight, you have to leave some things behind. For example, you have to let go of large food portions, lots of sweets and desserts, and dropping onto the couch instead of exercising.

Yes, you want to change! But even with the benefits of getting thinner, you probably miss the good times. That's grieving your progress. If you get stuck on missing the past, recognize you're holding onto a myth. You might remember that life was perfect. It wasn't. Or you convince yourself that if you could go back, you'd love it. You wouldn't.

Grieving what you've left behind is a healthy part of moving forward in life. Whether you lose a bunch of weight or go through challenging times, go ahead and grieve your progress.

Then find ways to replace the past and every day take steps in your new life. Climb the hill, drink your water and hold onto your goals. With time, the new you will become the best one!

TODAY

- Identify a life change or event that caused you to grieve your progress.

- Make a list of the losses or things you left behind with this event.

- Now create a list of ways you can replace those things in healthy ways.

ᔓ DAY 59 ᕙ
When there isn't enough

As I finished reading a bedtime story to Leah, my six-year-old niece, she said, "Do you really have to leave tomorrow? Can't you please stay a little longer?"

I told her I'd love to stay but I had to return home to go back to work. She started to cry and begged, "Are you sure you can't stay a few more days or maybe for another week?"

This was unusual behavior for Leah, and I wasn't sure how to respond. Leah's father had recently started work at a new job in another city and was coming home only once a month. The rest of the family was planning to move after school finished and their house was sold. As I looked at Leah's sad little face, I finally said, "You miss your daddy, don't you?"

"Oh yes," she responded. "I miss him a lot. I wish he was here tonight." Then I asked her, "Leah, if I stayed sitting on your bed all night, would that be long enough? Or if I stayed at your house for another week, would that be enough? Because I think you are missing your daddy, and no matter how long I stay, you will still wish he was here with you."

Leah nodded and tearfully admitted, "You're right. Even if you stayed here, my daddy would still be away. So I guess no matter how long you are at our house, it won't be enough. Until he gets home, I'll be feeling sad."

Your empty heart

There are a lot of times in life when you simply can't get enough. You yearn for more hugs, deeper conversations or appreciation for your work. When you don't get these things, you eat, hoping to fill the void. But it doesn't work because there isn't enough.

During these times, remember that food won't fix your empty heart. Instead, you have to identify what you need, then take care of those needs through nurturing and self-care activities.

Over time, you can become strong for whatever you face in your life. Even on days when you can't get enough love or comfort, you will be confident that you hold the power to your own nurturing. Inside your own spirit, there is enough!

TODAY

- Identify a recent time when you couldn't get enough of something you needed.

- Write a list of specific needs related to that time or event.

- Write a plan for how you can take care of your needs when there isn't enough.

∽ DAY 60 ∾
The gift of yourself

The two women in the restaurant booth next to me smiled a lot. Over cups of coffee and the senior breakfast special, they chatted quietly about many things. Clearly, they were good friends and companions for each other.

In spite of my efforts to avoid listening to their conversation, pieces of it slipped through. I soon realized that the woman with the flowing white hair asked a lot of questions, often repeating the same one they'd just finished discussing. But each time, her elderly friend quietly responded, using the same warm, caring voice as before.

Throughout the meal, she continued to speak sweetly to her white-haired friend, encouraging and supporting her in every way. When they got up to leave, she gently took her friend's elbow and guided her toward the door.

When I commented about these ladies to the staff, I learned that, every Monday, the woman picks up her forgetful friend and takes her out for breakfast, treating her with utmost love and respect, even on her worst memory days.

What a gift! These dear ladies reminded me again of the importance of kindness and patience in our world. Many times we get so wrapped up in our own struggles or frustrations that we forget how to encourage and support others.

Sharing your gift

Maybe you've fallen totally off your diet, or gone weeks without exercise. Perhaps you're discouraged because you've hit a plateau or regained some weight. I'm not suggesting these aren't important issues or that you ignore working on them.

But this week, maybe you could let go of fretting about yourself and your own weight-loss goals. Instead, focus on your ability to support and encourage others. Think about the words you need to hear, then give these words away to someone else.

There's something curious about giving encouragement. Even on your darkest days, sharing a tiny ray of hope with someone else will nearly always brighten your own spirit as well. This week, I challenge you to give support to everyone you meet. Seek out those who are troubled or feeling down, and share your gift by calling them or sending an encouraging note.

TODAY

- Find people who are trying to lose weight. Encourage them and tell them you know they can be successful. Describe their reactions.

- Send out five "I'm thinking of you" cards or "You can do it" emails.

- Record your thoughts about how it felt to share the gift of yourself.

DAYS 51–60 COMPLETED!

You've come this far in your 100 days...

Don't stop now. If you're struggling to stick with it, push yourself to finish *one more day*. You'll immediately be another day closer to achieving your weight-loss goals.

Just do one more day!

⤷ DAYS 61–70 ⤶

MANAGE EMOTIONS WITHOUT FOOD

‿ DAY 61 ‿
The emotional box

Remember how easily your emotions came when you were a child? Most of the time, you never questioned whether your emotions made sense—you just expressed what you felt.

But think about how you express your emotions now. Perhaps you rarely show anger and you certainly never cry. Instead of reacting when you feel sad or disappointed, you quietly push your thoughts aside and go on. In your mind, you believe you are in control of your feelings.

Emotions are connected

Unfortunately, emotions don't exist in isolation—they are all connected to the others. Picture a long cord with uncomfortable emotions such as anger, sadness, loneliness and boredom listed on the left end. The right end of the cord holds positive feelings such as love, happiness, sexuality and peacefulness.

When you pull in one side of the cord, the other side pulls in too. As you train yourself to never feel negative emotions such as anger and sadness, you also decrease your ability to feel positive ones such as true joy, peace and connection.

Living in the emotional box

If you block your emotions long enough, you can become so good at it that you stop feeling much of anything. You gradually build an invisible wall or an emotional box around yourself to keep your feelings inside at all times.

In this protected box, you continue to function as you always have. You go to work, you raise your children, you visit your mother. To the world, you look fine, but in truth, you've buried your authentic self.

Inside the box, you live in a neutral zone where you are emotionally dull. Without the ability to feel and express emotions, you disconnect yourself from life. Eventually, your zest for living slips away and intimate relationships become a chore.

What you don't realize is that food becomes necessary as a way to keep your emotions inside the box. So anytime you are tempted to allow an uncomfortable feeling, you eat something to push it back down.

Facing your emotions doesn't have to destroy you. When you take your feelings out of the dark, it makes them less scary. You may discover that your grief, anger, and even bitterness aren't as intense as you remembered.

TODAY

- Describe how you showed your emotions as a child. Did you laugh easily? Cry hard?

- Think about how you express emotions now. Describe how it's changed over the years.

- Identify common times when you eat instead of labeling or expressing your feelings.

∽ DAY 62 ∾
Revive my feelings

At a visit to my favorite coffee shop, I watched two women greet each other with a warm embrace. "I'm so sorry!" said one of the women. The second one quickly wiped her eyes and said, "Thanks. But I don't want to get all emotional. It feels too awful!"

I don't know what prompted her sadness. But as I watched the two friends, I noticed they each ate a large cinnamon roll along with their coffee. It appeared to work too, because I didn't see any more tears.

Eating instead of feeling

Looking at your feelings isn't always enjoyable. Emotions make you face the truth about life. Sometimes they force you to consider decisions or changes you may not be ready for. If your feelings make you too uncomfortable, you may try to escape them entirely.

But blocking your emotions also means you have to avoid certain thoughts. So you continue to ignore your disappointment with your marriage or your children. You pretend you enjoy working at a meaningless job that never challenges you. You push aside long-standing bitterness over your childhood or your current life path.

Food, of course, doesn't take away the true needs of your heart. It just puts a bandage on them, leaving them to fester under the surface until they spring back into your awareness. But sometimes, you keep eating because if you stop, you won't

136

make it through the day. And your weight keeps going higher because you can't bear to face your real life.

Reviving lost feelings

If you've lost touch with your emotions, you may need to pull some of them back to a conscious level. Recovering your feelings doesn't mean you have to start pounding your fists and screaming. You simply need to move out of the neutral zone and rebuild your enthusiasm for life.

As you explore ways to stop the patterns of emotional eating, you won't always like the solution. You may unearth pain you buried long ago, hoping never to face it again. And food will always lure you with the promise of an easy way to escape.

But don't ever give up on your efforts. When you don't require food to appease your emotions, staying on your diet and exercise program will become a whole lot easier.

TODAY

- Identify a situation where you might be using food to avoid difficult emotions.

- Consider ways to revive those emotions in healthy ways. Record your thoughts.

- Identify other places or situations where you try to avoid feeling, then create a plan for changing these patterns.

༄ DAY 63 ༄
What do I feel?

It's easy to think of emotions as being only three basic feelings: mad, sad and glad. But within each category are dozens of more specific words that describe how you might feel. Remember, your goal is to figure out what is driving your desire to eat.

Suppose you had a relationship break-up and feel depressed over it. Now consider more words that describe your present feelings. In addition to tearful and depressed, you might add lonely, discouraged and disappointed, all of which relate to the loss of the relationship.

I feel... because of...

Take a blank page of paper and draw a line down the middle from top to bottom. On the left side, write the words, "I feel," and on the right side write, "because of."

Choose a situation or event to explore and in the left column, write a word to describe how you feel about it. Then in the right column, add a reason or issue that prompted the emotion. For example, under "I feel..." you might write *angry*, and under "because of..." write *my partner doesn't help around the house.*

Keep this simple, using one or two words to identify each feeling and a short phrase or sentence to describe why you feel that way. Once you've written for a while, try to think of words that will help you be more accurate in describing how you feel.

If you're feeling angry, are you livid? Or are you bitter or overwhelmed? Perhaps your emotions are less intense, such as annoyed, irritated or simply grouchy? The more specific you can be, the greater your chance of doing something about your feelings instead of using food to appease them.

When you use the "I feel" exercise, you can write one or two feelings or make a list that fills an entire page. Take time to explore all the possible feelings related to the situation. You may discover many other emotions besides the intense feelings that showed up initially.

You don't even have to write the words down to be able to identify your feelings. You can just think them or even tell them to your steering wheel as you drive. Describing what you feel also helps decrease the intensity.

TODAY

- Identify a recent issue or situation that prompted a strong emotional reaction.

- Do the "I feel, because of" exercise and come up with several more emotion words.

- Choose the emotion that's most accurate, then write a plan for managing that emotion without reaching for food.

∾ DAY 64 ∾
Courage to feel

We don't have time to feel. We have to go to work, pick up kids, cook dinner, go visit our parents, attend a meeting. We certainly don't have time to cry.

Difficult emotions such as anger and grief can make you feel as if you are walking to the edge of a black hole where you can't see the bottom. You may be afraid that if you step into it, the pain will be unbearable.

You're afraid that if you start crying, you might not be able to stop. Or you worry that letting out your bitterness might cause you to explode and say mean, hurtful things.

Of course, to keep your feelings buried, you have to keep eating. So day after day, rather than give your emotions a chance to slip out, you use food to hold them in.

My own story

Despite years of intense efforts, my husband and I were not able to have children. I was born with an abnormally shaped uterus that can't support a full-term pregnancy. Three different times, I carried a pregnancy for six months before going into premature labor. Complications with the final pregnancy prevented me from ever being able to try again.

For many years, whenever I felt sad about my babies, I would eat a lot and try to avoid thinking. My weight-loss efforts never lasted because I spent so much time eating away the painful memories of losing my children.

One year after I'd battled an extensive winter depression, a counselor suggested I stop avoiding my emotions and allow myself to feel them instead. I was terrified by the thought, but I decided to follow her advice. It took a lot of courage, but with my counselor's help, I learned how to let my grief surface, then acknowledge it instead of eating to push it away. And I began to heal from my sadness.

Be willing to feel

If you want to be healthy about your emotions, you can't run from them. Instead, you have to be willing to sit with them and actually feel them. Sometimes this takes a lot of courage. But as I learned, it's the key to healing the pain and letting go of using food to keep it buried.

TODAY

- Describe a life issue where you avoid feeling emotion because it's painful.

- Use the exercise "I feel, because of" to label the feelings associated with this.

- Sit with the emotions and allow yourself to feel them and heal from them. Write about this experience.

∽ DAY 65 ∾
Showing emotions

During my childhood years, my parents kept the rules they'd each learned from their staunch German families. If you got mad, you could cry or yell quietly, but you couldn't throw things or hit anyone. People weren't supposed to hug or kiss in public. And you were to save the words, "I love you," for your life partner.

After years of watching my family rarely show emotions, I decided to become more open in demonstrating love and affection. So I made a plan for how I would show this to my parents by giving them hugs and telling them that I loved them.

I knew they might be uncomfortable with this, so I decided to teach them gradually how to show affection. My mother accepted my hugs quite readily, but getting a response from my father was a different story.

How I trained my father

When it was time for me to leave after one of my trips home, I waited until my father was standing beside my car. Then I reached up, put my arms around him in a cautious hug and said, "I love you, Daddy." He didn't move. He just stood there like a huge brick, with his hands firmly at his sides. Then he muttered, "Yeah, well, okay then. Have a safe trip."

On my next visit, I did this again, giving him a gentle hug when I left. This time, he reached up and briefly patted my arm. He still acted quite embarrassed, but he didn't back up or move away. Each time I went home, I would give him a hug and say, "I love you," even though he always acted stiff and uneasy.

As time went on, my father grew more comfortable with my show of affection. Eventually, he started reaching up and patting my shoulders when I hugged him. One day, almost two years after I'd started this little project, my father surprised me by gruffly saying, "I love you too." I was so moved by his unexpected response that I cried as I drove away.

Changing the way you show feelings doesn't have to be traumatic. You can start gradually, as I did, by expressing your emotions on a limited basis. Eventually, demonstrating your feelings will become easier and more enjoyable.

TODAY

- Describe a situation where you want to show your emotions.

- Make a plan for expressing your feelings. Describe the setting and what you'll do.

- When the time comes, carry out your plan. Write about how it worked.

❧ DAY 66 ❧
Kicking kettles

Some years ago, I went through a holiday season that was especially difficult. I missed my parents, who had both died in recent years. Other family members were far away, and our friends were busy or out of town. Because of a blizzard on Christmas Day, my husband and I decided to create a cozy holiday dinner at home.

With the salad made and the lasagna in the oven, we started cleaning up the kitchen. In our haste to get finished, we both shoved kettles into the cabinet at the same time, and my fingers got smashed between two iron pots.

The pain was awful! I was already an emotional wreck, and this pushed me over the edge. I sat down and started to cry. Although my fingers were throbbing, my heart seemed to hurt even more.

All I could think of was that I wanted to skip dinner and go eat a carton of ice cream. But as I headed for the freezer, my husband said, "I'm here, and it will be OK."

Those simple words caught my attention and I thought, "Wait a minute! Why am I letting some stupid iron pots make me eat ice cream?"

Suddenly, I turned back to the cupboard, then lifted my foot and kicked the offending kettle as hard as I could while I yelled, "Don't you EVER do that to me again!"

In that split second, my tears stopped and my emotions drained away. As I realized what I had done, I sank to the floor and melted into laughter. My husband sat down beside me, and we both laughed harder than we had in months.

A short while later, we lit the candles and enjoyed warm companionship over our wonderful holiday meal.

Blaming others

Kicking my kettles reminded me of how I tend to blame people, events or even iron pots for my eating struggles. During times when we're hurting or feeling weak and vulnerable, it's easy to think that eating will fix the problem. But food is only a temporary solution to your pain. The next day, the holes in your heart are still there.

So instead of reaching for ice cream or cookies during difficult times, pull out your tools for nurturing and self-care and make them a part of your day.

TODAY

- Recall a time when strong emotions made you want to eat.

- Identify the feelings that were prompting your desire for food.

- Create a short list of things you could have done instead of eating.

⮞ DAY 67 ⮜
Let it go

Ron's wife had an affair, then eventually left him for the other man. A short time later, she married her new boyfriend, and they seemed quite happy in their new life. As we talked, Ron described his intense sadness and depression over the loss of the relationship.

"I just can't get over it!" he said. "Lots of days, I still cry because I miss her so much. I know I'm overeating because I'm filling the void, but I just can't seem to get past this." When I asked Ron how long it had been since the relationship ended, he answered, "Nine years!"

To me, it didn't sound like Ron wanted to get over it. For one thing, his ongoing angst provided an excuse for his troubled eating. Ron's weight-loss efforts didn't work because he simply wasn't ready to let go of his hurt and anger.

Holding on serves a purpose

If you can't seem to let go of a feeling, consider the benefits of holding on to it. What keeps you attached to your sadness, anger or bitterness? What are you afraid will happen if you give it up?

Maybe you'll lose your ability to punish the other person. Perhaps you'd have to allow more intimacy or become accepting of a situation. If food provides a source of emotional comfort, you may unconsciously want to keep your negative feelings around.

I'll show you!

Years ago, Emily had a big fight with one of her sisters and couldn't seem to let go of her anger and bitterness. She kept thinking, "I'll show you! I'll make you understand how mean you are and prove that you can't treat me that way."

But Emily's anger didn't seem to harm her sister. It just kept Emily unhappy, and on days when the anger was especially strong, she would eat bags of chips as a way to "show her!" Emily's behavior was like holding a hot coal in your hand while saying, "I'll show you!" But who is the person getting burned?

Recognize areas where you are holding a hot coal, and make a conscious decision to let go of it. Work on healing your heart, and you'll probably find that eating to punish someone else will stop as well.

TODAY

- Identify a situation or event where you've had trouble letting go of your feelings.

- Consider the benefits of holding onto your anger, sadness or other emotions.

- Decide that it's time to let go of those feelings and heal your heart. Write about this.

✎ DAY 68 ✐

Guilt is not an emotion

"The day started out fine," Donna said. "I was following my diet plan like usual until someone brought chocolate triple layer cake into the office. I simply couldn't resist! First, I had a very small piece. Of course, the cake tasted wonderful. So I went back and got a larger piece, which I promptly devoured. Now I feel so guilty for giving in to the temptation. Sometimes, when I've messed up like that, I feel guilty for days!"

Is guilt an emotion?

When someone has committed a wrong act, the word *guilty* fits perfectly. You can be guilty of a crime or of cheating on your taxes or your spouse. But when you say you feel guilty around a non-criminal behavior, you are not describing a feeling.

Instead, the word *guilty* serves as a cover-up for a less acceptable emotion. When you peek underneath your guilty feelings, you may discover a whole list of emotions. The next time you feel guilty about something, ask yourself, "If I wasn't feeling guilty, what would I be feeling?"

Suppose, like Donna, you eat a piece of cake that wasn't on your diet plan. Maybe you feel disappointed because you couldn't resist a temptation or frustrated because you fell off your diet. You might feel embarrassed because your friends saw you eating the cake.

Perhaps you're afraid that you'll never lose weight or your spouse will yell at you. When you identify your real feelings, you recognize the insecurity and disappointment you would have missed if you hadn't looked beyond feeling guilty.

Feeling guilty about people

Cassie knew she should see her aging parents more often, but every time she returned home after visiting them, she went into an eating frenzy. She usually felt guilty about not visiting them sooner or not doing more things for them.

Cassie knew she also felt anger and frustration because of her parents' expectations and demands. She also began to realize she was devastated about their physical decline and worried about their future.

Instead of covering her thoughts by feeling guilty, she was able to identify and process what she really felt. Once she understood her emotions and shifted her attitude, Cassie was able to stop her eating binges.

TODAY

- Write down some times when you might say you feel guilty about something.

- Ask yourself, "If I wasn't feeling guilty, what would I be feeling?" Make a list.

- Decide how you can catch yourself using the word *guilty* and instead, identify your real feelings.

ꙮ DAY 69 ꙮ

Hurt feelings

At a recent dinner with friends, my husband made some comments that hurt my feelings. He thought he'd said them in fun, but I felt very embarrassed and humiliated by what he said.

Fortunately, we resolved this one pretty quickly. He admitted that he was exhausted from work and that when he's tired, he doesn't monitor his joking very well. Once we both understood how the conversation had come out differently than he'd intended, we were able to let it go and move on.

Someone breaks a rule

Most of us have mental rules for people's behaviors, and we expect others to talk or act in certain ways. When feelings get hurt, it's usually because someone broke one of these unspoken rules.

For example, I apparently have a rule that says my husband should not make jokes about me when we're with other people. Evaluate whether your rule makes sense or if you want to change it. If you choose to let go of your rule, you may find your hurt slips away almost immediately.

Healing your hurt

When hurt feelings linger, they can pull you down into sadness or disappointment. And sometimes, the anger that goes with the hurt can make you unwilling to let go of it very easily.

Feeling hurt harms your trust as well as your sense of emotional safety. You might feel violated or disillusioned that someone would treat you that way. You may shake your head in amazement or disbelief and think, "How could they do this to me?"

During these times, a carton of ice cream or a bag of cookies can look pretty appealing. Food seems to help us nurse the hurt for a while. And for some reason, we don't usually reach for a salad or a bunch of carrots for this activity!

Regardless of what caused them, hurt feelings are valid. They typically represent some type of loss, and it's important that you allow yourself to feel sadness or grief. So go ahead and cry.

Express your feelings of letdown or despair. In your journal, write about your disappointments and the reasons behind them. Then instead of reaching for food as a way to heal, figure out ways you can let the feelings go and take care of your heart.

TODAY

- Think of a time, either recent or in the past, when your feelings were hurt.

- Identify the unspoken rule that was broken. Does that rule make sense?

- Write about how you can heal the hurt feelings and let them go.

∾ DAY 70 ∾

Eating instead of thinking

Lynn and her twin brother had always been close. When he died in a car accident, she had a hard time coping with the loss. Because she didn't want to let her memories come to the surface, she avoided thinking about them for years.

She said, "After my brother died, I couldn't bear feeling my grief. It was like I stored my emotions in a box with a lid. Whenever I tried to lose weight, the box would peek open and the feelings of loss would pop out. So I'd eat until I shoved the lid back down. I finally realized that before I could be successful with losing weight, I had to deal with my grief and my emotional pain."

Like my experience with losing pregnancies, eating allows you to escape emotions you can't bear to think about. Eating a whole pizza or another piece of chocolate cake can shove even the most painful feelings deep inside. And when you bury your negative emotions, you can pretend you are over them or even deny they existed.

Feeling is painful

Often we keep our difficult feelings buried because we can't face the pain of dealing with them. So when sadness or bitterness creep to the surface, we quickly eat more, shoving the feelings back down where they no longer can hurt us.

Overeating also keeps us from facing the realities of our lives. Ann realized that she was using her weight as an excuse for her life problems. She said, "As long as I feel lousy about my weight, I can avoid looking at what could actually be making me feel that way in my life.

"I can concentrate on points, measurements, and food lists and never touch the real issues. That way I don't actually have to deal with my awful job, my lousy marriage or other issues that are affecting me."

Even though it can be very painful, it's time to take the lid off the box and allow yourself to see what's there. Once you allow yourself to think about the pain in your life, you will become more willing to feel it. With time, you'll experience healing and peace instead of eating to push your feelings away.

TODAY

- Identify an issue or event you don't want to think about that might be causing eating struggles.

- Plan a time to sit with your thoughts about this issue and allow yourself to feel the emotions that come up.

- Record your insights as well as your ideas on how to deal with this issue instead of eating.

DAYS 61–70 COMPLETED!

You've come this far in your 100 days...

Don't stop now. If you're struggling to stick with it, push yourself to finish *one more day*. You'll immediately be another day closer to achieving your weight-loss goals.

Just do one more day!

✌ DAYS 71–80 ❧

OVERCOME BARRIERS AND SABOTAGE

❧ DAY 71 ❧
Setback or failure?

Some years ago, I fell while walking my dog and ended up with a painful bruised rib. As days went by, I gradually began to heal. But my spirit took a nosedive. I had worked hard to build up my exercise program and suddenly I couldn't do any of it.

I felt like a failure. To console myself, I slid into eating ice cream and cookies. Of course, that comforted me for a little while, but then I felt worse because I was unhappy about my eating.

Finally, I decided I'd coped long enough and I was ready to get back on track with my weight-management efforts. I also realized I had to change my viewpoint and label this time as a setback, not a failure.

Sometimes a difficult loss, such as the death of a parent or the end of a relationship, will cause you to go through a setback. But at other times, you can struggle because of simple things such as tripping on the sidewalk.

Whether you are dealing with grief or a sprained ankle, a setback can make you lose your motivation and cause you to temporarily give up on your weight-loss plan.

Allow a recovery period
Overcoming a setback doesn't have to take a long time. Start by giving yourself a recovery period. Cry as much as you want. Pound your frustration out on your pillow or a punching bag. Be angry or discouraged or depressed.

When you're ready to move on again, you will know it. At that point, your recovery period is over, and you need to choose to get back on track.

Return to what worked.

Make a list of things that have worked for you in the past, including any routines or activities that help you stay committed to your goals. Pull out your tracking notebook or sign in to your online program. Review your list of reasons why you want to lose weight and remind yourself that you really do care about your goals and your health.

A setback doesn't have to ruin your weight-loss efforts. Instead of considering it a disaster, view a setback as a gift. Let it be a time of learning and renewal, rather than a dent in your belief that you can be successful.

TODAY

- Recall a time when you've had a setback. Write about how you handled it.

- Create a setback plan you can pull out quickly when you need it.

- Pretend you've had a setback, then start using your new plan. Record your thoughts.

✣ DAY 72 ✣
Renew your vision

When I was in school for my master's degree, I once registered for a class that would meet all day Saturday and Sunday. As I began gathering my textbooks and notepads the day before the first session, I realized I felt totally overwhelmed and almost sick with exhaustion.

I thought, "I'm so tired that I can't see how I'll be able to make it through the class." Finally, I built up my courage and called the professor.

As soon as she answered the phone, I started to cry. "I just can't do this!" I said. "I'm physically and emotionally exhausted, and even though I need this class, I can't see how to push through my fatigue and be there for the entire weekend."

"Then don't," she said.

I wasn't sure I'd heard her right. I'd expected a pep talk in which she'd push me to do what was required to finish my program. But in her warm, gentle style, she continued, "Linda, I know you're committed to getting your degree, and missing this class won't change that.

"So instead of forcing yourself to go this weekend, I want you to relax and take care of yourself. Eventually, you'll have to replace it with some other course, but right now, you need to allow some time for renewal. View this weekend as a gift and let it strengthen your commitment to your program."

Build your vision

What an interesting idea! Using a challenge as a way to strengthen commitment! During that weekend, I spent time resting as well as renewing my determination to finish my studies. I also thought about my vision of walking across the stage at graduation and receiving my degree. And when that day came, I knew it was because I had stayed committed, even during the setbacks.

In your weight-loss efforts, always hold a vision of the outcome you want. Imagine having more energy, moving easier and enjoying better health. Picture easily sliding into an airline seat or getting up off the floor from playing with your kids or grandkids.

Let these images sustain you, even during times when you take a break to rest and recover. Renew your vision over and over and use it to strengthen your commitment to achieving your weight-loss goals.

TODAY

- Create a vision page in your notebook. Add images and words that show the outcomes you want.

- Describe how you will feel when you reach these outcomes.

- Review your vision at the end of the day and record your response to it.

✎ DAY 73 ✎
Manage special days

Although she was newly single, Sarah didn't think that Valentine's Day would be a problem this year. But something went wrong. "I don't know what happened," she said. "I bought myself flowers and I made a list of non-food activities that I love. Then I picked out a couple of them to do on Valentine's Day."

But on the way home from work, Sarah stopped at the grocery store for a take-out salad. There she saw a huge display with all the Valentine's Day chocolates at half price. Because she can't resist a good bargain, she grabbed two boxes, thinking she could save them for a later time. But that didn't work either.

She said, "As soon as I got home, I opened a box and ate one of the chocolates. Soon I reached for another piece and then a couple more. Instead of eating my healthy salad, I finished off the entire box of candy and half of the second one before I came to my senses. What is wrong with me?"

"There's nothing wrong with you," I replied. "It sounds like you needed a friend, and that box of candy did a fine job of spending time with you. But here's an idea. Let's mentally create the day exactly as you had wanted it. Pretend that Valentine's Day went perfectly, then write down the things you would have done instead."

Sarah's perfect day

Sarah thought about what would have made the holiday go better, and here's what she came up with:

- Plan ahead for dinner and put a meal in the slow cooker before leaving for work. That way I'll have something to look forward to when I get home.
- Skip the grocery store on holidays. If I don't see the candy, I won't be tempted by the discount price.
- As soon as I get home, get on my treadmill and exercise for 15 to 20 minutes. That usually helps me stay determined to take care of myself the rest of the evening.

Sarah was excited. "This feels way more positive than analyzing my mistakes." Then she paused for a second. "I better get out my slow-cooker recipe book this week. Easter is coming, and I already know where the store will display the chocolate bunnies!"

TODAY

- Look at the calendar and identify the next special holiday that will include food temptations.

- Write a list of three things you will do to manage that day when it comes.

- Create a reminder note for your plan and put it on the calendar or on your phone. Record what you did.

✎ DAY 74 ❧
It's not my fault

Wouldn't it be nice if being overweight wasn't really your fault? You could simply tell people you have a weight problem because your mother (or boyfriend or boss) always insists that you eat. Maybe you're right. Do you ever hear any of these comments?

- What's the matter, don't you like my food? I thought this was your favorite.
- I made this cherry pie just for you. What do you mean, you don't want any?
- Come on, everyone else is eating. Besides, we have to celebrate!

Most of us don't like conflict, so when someone tells us to eat, we do it. Or we get caught up in pleasing others, even though it might cause us to overeat. We also know resisting could mean we'll have to deal with people acting insulted or feeling hurt.

Pam told me, "Whenever I fell off my diet, I'd always blame other people, such as my friends or my family. I convinced myself they were the reason I failed. Finally I realized that no one was going to do this for me. Instead of blaming others, I had to face my own problems and figure out how to make my plan work."

No one can make you follow a healthy eating or exercise plan, so it's up to you to manage these areas of your life. Weight-loss success happens when you take charge of your own goals instead of counting on other people.

Be a *broken record*

Using a broken record approach helps you wear people down when they are pushing you to eat. Just keep saying the same phrase or some variation of it over and over. For example, whenever someone offers you food, just say, "Not just yet, I'm going to wait a little while."

You can use this line repeatedly at parties or gatherings, and most people will never realize you didn't eat during the entire event. It provides a gracious way to manage the discomfort of being pushed when you don't want to eat.

If someone returns or offers you food again, simply repeat the phrase or a variation of it. The "I'll wait until later" response can help you stay strong any time you feel pressured to take seconds or eat dessert.

TODAY

- Identify situations where you tend to blame others for your eating struggles.

- Write about how you can manage these times instead of eating to please others.

- Come up with several phrases to use for a "broken record" response when people push you to eat. Write them down.

❧ DAY 75 ❧
The people hook

Every time Marilyn started a new diet plan, someone would have a crisis. She kept hoping her children would grow up and take care of their own lives. But they didn't. And whenever they had problems, Marilyn not only rushed in to help, she ate.

Marilyn believed she was being a concerned and caring parent. But she also struggled with saying "no" to other people in her life, such as her mother and her boss. In reality, she had become so hooked into other people's lives that she had no concept of her own identity.

Marilyn had become a victim of the people hook. Other people and their problems constantly pulled her into feeling distraught, worried and upset. At the same time, she also got hooked into trying to fix all of their dilemmas.

When you become overly involved in other people's lives, you eventually become so lost in other people's problems that your own self-esteem and confidence fade away. Perhaps you assume that after all you've done for them, people will give back to you or show you more love. Unfortunately, you seldom get the payback you hoped for.

Soon you start feeling resentful because people you've helped don't appreciate it and they simply take you for granted. When you don't get the gratitude or attention you anticipated, it's easy to try to find it in food.

Time to get unhooked

Look carefully at whether people hooks are driving your emotional eating. You can still care about the people you love. Just don't let yourself disappear in the process. Remember this important guideline: It's not your job to fix people. It's your job to love them!

If you feel like you've lost yourself as a result of taking care of others, you may have to make some hard choices around the people in your life. This may mean allowing them to manage their lives without your constant help.

When your friends or family members call with another dilemma, decide how you can contribute and when you need to back off. Encourage people around you to take responsibility for themselves. And learn to say no more often instead of always trying to keep everybody happy.

TODAY

- Identify places in life where you get caught in the people hook.

- Create a plan that will help you unhook and say no when needed.

- Make a sign that says: "It's not my job to fix them. It's my job to love them."

∾ DAY 76 ∾
Stop sabotaging me

Kim worked hard at her weight-loss program and dropped nearly 150 pounds. As her energy and confidence improved, she began to speak up for herself and her own needs. Gradually, her husband realized he was losing his power over her and he wasn't entirely happy with her new life.

She said, "At Christmas last year, he gave me a huge box of chocolates and a beautiful blouse, size 4X. However, at this point, I was wearing a size 12 and the blouse was enormous on me.

"After I opened my gifts, he hugged me and said he wanted the old Kim back. What he really wanted was the woman who was totally dependent on him for everything, including getting compliments, attention and affection."

When you feel sabotaged

When it's clear that your support people are getting in the way of your progress, try to determine what makes them feel so uncomfortable. Are they acting out of ignorance because they actually don't know how to give support? Or could they be harboring deeper feelings such as a fear of losing their power over you?

Friends or family members may worry about losing a partying buddy or the person they can always count on for sharing a pizza. Jackie's boyfriend kept dishing up two bowls of ice cream every night. He seemed to "forget" that she was trying to lose weight.

To counteract sabotaging behaviors, assure people that you will continue to love and appreciate them, even though you are making changes in your life. Let them know you value their relationships and that you will continue to want to spend time with them.

Help people recognize behaviors that sabotage you and tell them what you need instead. For example, ask your kids to close bags of chips or cookies and put them in a cupboard instead of leaving them on the counter. Tell your friends you still want to go out with them but you will be ordering different food and drinks than in the past.

Once your family or friends realize they are still important to you, they may stop fretting about what you are doing. If these efforts don't work, ignore their comments or avoid certain people until you feel more confident about your progress.

TODAY

- Notice how people are reacting to you and what they are saying. Write about areas where you feel sabotaged.

- Plan a time to talk to them about your needs and write out what you will say.

- Record the responses of the people you talked with.

❦ DAY 77 ❦
My sabotage toolbox

Sabotage can happen anywhere, even with people you don't even know. Maybe you've had a server at a restaurant say, "Is that all you're going to eat? Didn't you like it?" Or the host of a party will keep pushing you to eat more because it's homemade cheesecake.

These people don't want to harm your weight-loss efforts. They usually don't even realize they might be sabotaging you. Even good friends or family members can forget that you are working so hard to stay on your weight-loss program.

But if you are vegetarian and someone offers you a piece of shrimp, you don't suddenly become a meat eater. You simply say, "No, thank you," and go back to your own plate.

In the same way, it's your job to manage situations where you are dealing with food pushers. Instead of feeling angry or frustrated at the potential saboteurs, keep a mental toolbox of tricks you can pull out at a moment's notice. Here are some things to include in your toolbox.

Use the magic phrase

Anytime you feel pressured to eat something not on your diet, tell the food pusher, "Not just yet. I'm going to wait a little while." If they ask again, just repeat this phrase or some variation of it. "Thanks, but I'll still wait a bit." Because it appears you'll eat eventually, people will usually leave you alone.

Don't talk about it

Avoid troublesome diet discussions by saying, "My weight-loss counselor said I shouldn't talk about my program because it makes me want to eat." This prevents revealing details about your plan or the amount of weight you've lost.

Blame your doctor

Say things such as, "My doctor has me on a special food plan right now because of my stomach (or heart, cholesterol.) So I'm sorry, but I'll need to avoid a couple of things in this meal."

Sabotage happens only if you allow it. Even if someone is intentionally trying to make you slip up, stay strong and committed to your plan. Remember that your goals are more important than pleasing others. Remind yourself that you are determined to live at a healthy weight and that you value that outcome more than being part of a crowd.

TODAY

- Watch for people or situations that might sabotage your efforts. Record what you notice.

- Choose a response you will feel comfortable saying when this happens. Write it down, then practice saying it out loud.

- Record what happens when you use this response to avoid sabotage.

❧ DAY 78 ❧
Self-sabotage

Suzanne was frustrated with her progress. She told me, "I've lost 54 pounds and have just reached 195 on the scale. But I keep bouncing back up over 200. I have 40 more pounds to go to be at my goal. I can't figure out why I keep sabotaging my success. It's almost like I don't want to reach my goal."

Self-sabotage can stem from a lot of different things. Maybe you don't think you deserve to be thin or you worry that it will be too hard to maintain a lower weight. Perhaps losing weight is too scary or you don't feel confident or comfortable as a thin person.

Sometimes it takes a lot of soul-searching to figure out what's really in your way of being at a healthier weight. You may need to ask yourself some hard questions about what's keeping you from being successful. It's not easy or a lot of fun to do this but it's a critical part of your journey.

Weight as protection

Soon after Mary Ann reached her goal weight of 160 pounds, she went to a party where she was attacked and raped. During her healing and recovery time, she gained back a lot of weight. In her efforts to lose weight again, every time she got close to the weight she was at when she was harmed, she would go off her plan and eat her way back up to 200 pounds.

As we explored the barriers around reaching her goals, it became clear that body memories made her fearful that

170

something bad would happen to her again when she got close to her goal weight.

Sometimes people who sabotage themselves have an unconscious need to stay overweight. If you've been a victim of rape, incest or other abusive behavior, your weight may be helping you feel safe. Your size can also protect you from getting involved in relationships or facing the prospect of physical intimacy.

Overcoming self-sabotage requires building a trust that you will be strong and safe at any weight. Mary Ann eventually took a kickboxing class that gave her confidence she could protect herself from harm and be successful at reaching her goals. In your own life, work on self-talk and inner power that will help you trust yourself at any weight.

TODAY

- Identify places in life where you might be sabotaging yourself.

- Make a list of things you are fearful of or that might not be good when you reach your goal weight.

- Plan ways to manage each of the things on your list.

⤴ DAY 79 ⤵
Rebellion

Gina was ready to give up on losing weight. She said, "I feel like I am being controlled by a bratty inner child that wants to do whatever she feels like. Today I caught myself eating treats someone brought to work. I quit once I saw what I was doing, but later I ate more and they weren't even that good."

Gina told me she was feeling a lot of anger and resentment about dieting. She was aware she was sabotaging herself, but she was angry she couldn't have foods she wanted and eat whatever she felt like.

"I'm so tired of having to watch everything I eat and pay attention to every detail. I'm angry that I'm supposed to exercise and not keep cookies in my home. And I'm really sick of thinking about food and craving it all the time. Eventually I just rebel and decide to eat as much as I want of those cookies and chips."

I thought for a minute, then asked Gina, "So how is rebellion working for you? Is it making you happy or peaceful in life?"

"Of course not!" she said. "It makes me feel miserable, and it's made my weight get higher than ever. I guess it's time to stop rebelling, but I don't know how to do that."

Who am I?

Over the next months, Gina and I began working on changing her identity from a rebellious child to a healthy adult. I asked her, "Where is your identity right now? Do you see yourself as a strong, vibrant, healthy woman? One who manages stress, challenges, conferences and social events without needing food as a coping solution?

"Or do you still see yourself as an overweight, depressed woman who always fails at managing her weight? Because that's how you seem to be living."

A lot of Gina's struggles were related to her weak self-esteem and lack of believing in herself. She admitted she didn't like living the way she was. She also realized she was tired of thinking a food craving was more important than having a healthy body.

I challenged Gina to let go of her negative identity and start viewing herself as a positive, successful, healthy woman. It wasn't easy, but over time, she was able to do this and was successful at reaching her goals.

TODAY

- Write about times you rebel or feel resentful in your weight-loss efforts.

- Define your positive identity with words such as *strong, vibrant* and *healthy*.

- Live in that identity today and record how it changes your behaviors.

ꙮ DAY 80 ꙮ
Too comfortable

Darcy was upset about constantly falling off her weight-loss plan. She told me, "Some days I just don't care about working on it. It's so much easier to just let it go." Unfortunately, Darcy's extra 60 pounds were affecting her health as well as her energy. But she admitted she wasn't very desperate and that staying the same felt much easier than changing.

Perhaps you have a similar viewpoint. You like being able to eat whatever you want, flop into the recliner after work and sip a cold beer. You are simply "too comfortable" and don't feel like pushing yourself to lose weight.

Occasionally you whine about your miserable situation, but you don't do anything different. When you think about starting a weight-loss plan and staying with it, you put off deciding for a while. Of course, by avoiding a decision, you've already made your choice—to stay the same.

Fear drives it

Being too comfortable is often related to a sense of fear. What if you fail again, repeating the embarrassing weight regain you've done in the past? What if you aren't strong enough to stay on a weight-loss plan until you reach your goal? Worst of all, what if you aren't happy once you get there?

Rather than face these fears and overcome them, you may slide into not caring or not making any effort to change. But are you really comfortable? Do you have this nagging thought that you're afraid of what will happen if you don't change?

Hitting bottom

Perhaps you believe you have to "hit bottom" before you will do something. When will that happen and how will you know when you hit it? Perhaps you are there now. It's all in how you define it.

In his book, *Getting Unstuck*, Dr. Sidney Simon defines bottom as "the moment you decide you want to be happier, healthier, more creative, successful or fulfilled than you already are."

You don't have to go through a health crisis or a dramatic event to hit bottom. Instead, you can create your own version of it right now. Make this the moment you decide to change your life and your future. Then start taking steps to move past your comfort level, knowing it will bring you to the outcome you really want.

TODAY

- List the fears you have about dieting or losing weight.

- Label today as the day you "hit bottom." Write about what that feels like.

- Describe what actions you'll take today to move yourself past being too comfortable.

DAYS 71–80 COMPLETED!

You've come this far in your 100 days...

Don't stop now. If you're struggling to stick with it, push yourself to finish *one more day*. You'll immediately be another day closer to achieving your weight-loss goals.

Just do one more day!

❧ DAYS 81–90 ❧

DEAL WITH EMOTIONAL CHALLENGES

☙ DAY 81 ❧
Problem or predicament

When my father's health was declining, I worried about him but couldn't visit easily because I lived too far away. So I decided to send him a card once a week. Some were funny, while others were more serious but warm and caring. I always wrote a few lines in the cards and signed them with "Love you."

After my father passed away, I was visiting my family one weekend and my mom handed me a large shoebox. She said, "I thought you might like to see this." Inside the box were all the cards that I'd sent to my father. According to my mom, he'd read many of them over and over, and always felt closer to me as a result of those cards.

Is this a predicament or a problem?

Counseling psychologist Dr. Paul Welter divides stress-related issues into two major types: predicaments and problems. He defines a predicament as a stressful situation that won't change for a long time, or in some cases, may never change.

Having a bad job or a troubled marriage is a predicament. So are financial problems, being overweight or raising teenagers. In each of these situations, all you can do is wait for time to pass and hope the predicament will improve or end.

Action plans

Instead of getting overwhelmed by a predicament, Dr. Welter suggests breaking it down into smaller components or problems. Once you have a list of problems, you can take action steps to work on them.

For example, my father's illness was a predicament, but feeling disconnected from him was a problem. And my action step created a wonderful way for me to connect with him and show him my love.

With the predicament of being overweight, problems might include eating fast-food meals on workdays or not taking time to exercise. With each problem, you can create an action plan that will help you manage it differently. For example, you might decide to bring your own lunch and to join a health club so you can fit exercise in more easily.

Instead of wasting energy or eating over situations that aren't going to change, learn to identify the problems inside a predicament. With each of those problems, take action in places where it will make a difference.

TODAY

- Identify a couple of predicaments in your life that won't change quickly.

- Below each predicament, figure out a few specific problems.

- Create action steps for each problem. Put some of them in place today.

ॐ DAY 82 ॐ
Whose problem is it?

Late one afternoon, Helen's daughter called and said her babysitter had cancelled at the last minute. Because she didn't want her daughter to miss work at her evening job, Helen drove over to her daughter's home and bailed her out.

But over the next few months, her daughter kept having last-minute challenges with not being able to get a sitter or having one cancel on short notice. Even though she was often exhausted from her own job and other commitments, Helen kept going over and helping her daughter out.

In our discussions, Helen told me she wasn't making any progress with her weight-loss goals because she kept eating snacks along with her daughter's young children. But she also knew that her exhaustion was contributing to her bad eating patterns.

I asked Helen, "Whose problem is it that your daughter doesn't have a regular babysitter right now?" Helen thought, then answered, "I guess it's her problem."

"That's right," I responded. "It's her problem. And do you want to make it yours?"

"No, I absolutely don't," she said. The next day, Helen had a talk with her daughter and informed her that she was going to be unavailable for babysitting for the next couple of months, and maybe even longer.

Her daughter squirmed a bit and tried to get Helen to change her mind. But it soon became clear that her daughter had to take care of her own problem and find new babysitters.

Two questions

Are you constantly fixing something that isn't your problem? If so, it's time to make a decision that you'll stop taking care of the world. Any time you struggle with getting too involved with other people's issues, ask yourself these two questions:

1. Whose problem is it?
2. Do I want to make it mine?

If you conclude that you do not want to make it your problem, let go of your involvement. When you make a decision to stop trying to fix things that aren't your problem, you'll feel a sense of relief. You'll also be less likely to head for the refrigerator every time the problem comes back up.

TODAY

- Watch for a situation where you can ask the questions in this lesson. Describe it.

- If you conclude it's not your problem, plan how you will let go of your involvement.

- Record what happened after you stopped making that problem yours.

❧ DAY 83 ❧
No one takes care of me

Jenny knew her mother wasn't able to give her much nurturing anymore, but she couldn't figure out how to replace it. She said, "One Saturday, I decided to visit my aging mother, who was in declining health. On the way to her home, I stopped at my favorite bakery and picked up a couple of large chocolate chip cookies.

"When I bit into one of those soft, chewy cookies, I was instantly overwhelmed by some of the most intense emotions I have ever felt. It was as though every part of my body suddenly filled with deep feelings of love and comfort. I don't understand why they affected me this much but the feelings were so powerful that I began to sob."

When Jenny thought about what happened, she realized the cookies reminded her of how her mother had always loved her and taken care of her. As her mother's health and mental ability faded, so did her nurturing role. Jenny said, "Since Mom can't take care of me anymore, I let food do it instead. I can't seem to stop eating those cookies because they replace the only way I felt nurtured and loved."

Feeling alone

What do you do when your emotional support slips away? When you go through a divorce or other relationship changes, you can lose the connections that nurtured you and made you feel emotionally safe. You can also experience this with an aging parent or other changes to family members.

Like Jenny, you may have lost a relationship that provided nurturing or comfort. Until you rebuild these missing areas of your life, you risk using food to replace them.

Often we keep our difficult feelings buried because we can't face the pain of dealing with them. So when sadness or bitterness creeps to the surface, we quickly eat more, shoving the feelings back down where they no longer can hurt us.

Do you have areas in life where you have lost emotional support? Time helps heal this, but you also have to create new ways to feel nurtured and cared for. This takes effort as well as energy, but it's critical to recovering from your loss. Don't give up. Eventually the pain will heal and your ability to cope without eating will return.

TODAY

- Identify a place in your life where you have lost emotional support or comfort.

- Write about what has changed in your life because of that loss.

- Create at least two ideas for taking care of your needs for emotional support.

❧ DAY 84 ❧
Body memories

It happens once a year. My exercise program goes away and I find myself eating a lot more cookies, desserts and nighttime ice cream. For a long time, I couldn't figure out why I would slide into this pattern. Although things seemed fine, I would feel off balance and sort of "out of sync" with life.

When I described this feeling to my friend, she asked, "When was your dog, Peppy, born?" I thought for a minute, then said, "She was born on March 30th, so she's almost seven years old."

"That's it," my friend said quietly. "Remember what else happened that day? I think you're having a body memory and it's pulling you down, causing you to overeat."

As soon as she said it, I knew! That was the same day I got the dreaded call from my doctor telling me I had breast cancer. Tears slipped out as I remembered that very difficult time in my life. Memories flooded back about the surgery, oncologists and medications with terrible side effects.

Fortunately, I've made it past all of that, and I'm celebrating many years of being a breast cancer survivor. But I realize that each year, anticipation of that date was leading me into the cupboards and the refrigerator.

Recognize it

Body memories happen all the time. You hear a song on the radio and suddenly remember your senior prom or the pain of divorce or other losses. Often, we don't recognize we're having a body memory. We just see the symptoms of overeating, not exercising and feeling out of sync.

When you can't figure out what's causing a change in your eating and exercise patterns, look at the calendar or your journal. Are you coming up on the anniversary of a traumatic time or the loss of someone you loved?

Often body memories will remind you of the event long before your brain does. And many times, anticipation of the memory causes more struggle than the actual anniversary or event. In my own life, I've learned to recognize when I'm having a body memory. Then I remind myself to do extra nurturing and self-care to get through that challenging time.

TODAY

- Identify a place or situation when a body memory might affect you or tempt you to eat.

- Write about the event or loss that prompts a body memory. Allow yourself to feel sadness or other emotions this brings up.

- Make a short list of ways to comfort yourself instead of reaching for food to cope.

✑ DAY 85 ✑
Dealing with grief

L ynn had been thinking that life was good. But just as she turned onto her street, the radio began playing an old Michael Bolton song that pushed open her memory bank.

Although it had been five years since her husband died, hearing that song brought a crushing pain into Lynn's chest. A tear slid down her cheek, followed by another. The moment she pulled her car into the garage, she buried her head on the steering wheel and sobbed.

Finally, she stopped crying and tried to pull herself together. As she stumbled into the house, she thought, "What's wrong with me? I should be over this by now!"

In reality, no matter how much time passes, you'll never be completely over a devastating loss. Even after you've moved on, you'll always carry some leftover grief in your heart.

The healing road

When you grieve a loss, you move gradually down a healing road. To understand this process, imagine a long path with sections representing the amount of healing you've accomplished so far.

Begin by picturing the time you experienced the loss, followed by the early days of agony and emotional pain. After those initial weeks, you began inching forward until you reached a healing level of 10 or 20 percent. As time passed, you continued to move slowly through more sections of healing.

At the 80 percent mark, you might have felt like much of your grief is behind you. But this is where you stopped because the final 20 percent is where you hold memories. It also represents the love and meaning you originally felt in the relationship or situation, even if it was years ago.

It's that last 20 percent that makes you choke up, even years later, when you see a forgotten photo or hear a favorite song on the radio. In other words, you never get over it completely.

Knowing you don't ever have to be done with grief gives you a tremendous sense of freedom. Eventually, that 20 percent may open up less often. But when it does show up, don't fight your feelings. Instead of pushing to get past them and forget your loss, remind yourself those memories are part of your healing.

TODAY

- Identify a time you've been through the loss of a person or even a pet. Describe how you felt at the time of the loss.

- Picture the healing road and identify some of the sections you've gone through.

- Write about the memories that will always remain in your last 20 percent of healing.

❧ DAY 86 ❧
Talk to the bear

When my husband arrived at the hospital, he brought me a fluffy, white teddy bear with a navy bow around its neck. As we drove home, he asked if I wanted to stop for breakfast. But I couldn't speak. So I simply nodded. In the quiet restaurant, I sat clutching the little white bear, never letting go even through several cups of coffee and a cheese omelet.

A few days earlier, a tubal pregnancy had put me into emergency surgery and eliminated my chance to ever have a baby. My heart was breaking, and I also felt sad for my husband. But no matter how I tried, I couldn't get any words to come out of my mouth.

Finally, I began talking to the little white bear. "It's okay," I said. "We're going to make it. We both feel sad and we don't know what to do. But we've been through hard times before, and we'll get through this one too." The bear just sat there, serenely loving back with the comfort and acceptance a teddy bear gives.

During the weeks that followed, I had many conversations with that teddy bear. Little by little, I felt the pain ease in my heart and knew I was starting to heal. That little bear helped me survive feeling more raw and discouraged than I ever remembered.

Teddy bear as therapist
Strange as it sounds, you can actually use a teddy bear or other stuffed animal to help you heal. Instead of keeping

thoughts and sadness inside, you can share them with this friend.

Start by choosing a favorite stuffed animal or doll to use as your friend. Place it on a chair or stool in front of you, then start talking out loud. Describe what you're thinking and feeling today. Cry if you want. Your friend will continue to listen with great empathy and caring.

If you prefer, hold the friend on your lap and feel the comfort of connecting with it. During your visit, write some notes about your thoughts and insights. Do this once or twice a week and let your friend help you move forward in your healing.

TODAY

- Choose a favorite stuffed animal to talk to about your thoughts and feelings.

- Plan a time when you can be alone and have a visit with this friend.

- Sit with the friend and talk through anything you wish. It might be related to a loss, but could also be about current frustrations or needs. Record how that went.

❧ DAY 87 ❧
Allow a grace period

For two years, Barb watched her mother's health decline. When her mom's condition reached a point where she could no longer live alone, Barb helped her downsize from her rural home and move into an assisted living center.

Most days, Barb drove 25 miles to spend time with her mom, bringing her gifts and reading books aloud to her and a group of residents at the center. But as the months went by, her mom's illness got worse and eventually she passed away.

Throughout this time of watching her mother's decline, Barb kept trying to lose weight. We spent a lot of our coaching sessions working on motivation and inner strength. But the drain on Barb's spirit during this time was awful, and she kept slipping up on her weight-loss plan. At the time of her mother's death, Barb's weight was higher than before her mom became ill.

Healing takes time

As a coach, I wondered if I should I have pushed Barb harder to stay on her program. But during this time, especially the last months of her mother's life, I realized Barb needed to allow herself a grace period.

That meant giving herself a break and not expecting perfection in her efforts. We talked a lot about improving her ability to nurture and care for herself, even during the painful last days of her mom's life.

Since her mother's death, Barb has done a lot of healing. But we allowed the grace period to continue until she felt it was the right time for losing weight again. Finally she was ready and she began a new weight-loss plan that gave her wonderful progress.

Managing a grace period

A grace period doesn't mean you throw away healthy eating and give up on exercise. You still need to pay attention to those things. But it's also a time to minimize the damage or take walks that last only ten minutes.

Labeling a tough time as a grace period allows you to be forgiving when you aren't perfect or you slip back into eating cookies. When it's time to move out of the grace period, you'll recognize it. At that point, you'll be ready to return to a healthy path and start moving forward again.

TODAY

- Identify a recent or even long-ago time when you needed a grace period.

- Write about what it would have been like to forgive yourself and allow grace during this time.

- Consider how you can apply this to any current or recent situation. Record this.

～ DAY 88 ～
Junk in the backyard

When you have painful memories around certain life events, you can become obsessed with figuring out how to heal from them. If you believe you have to get over these things before you can make progress in other areas, you may never reach your goals.

Instead of dwelling on painful memories, learn how to acknowledge your past, then let it go. To do this, picture yourself living in a small house with a fenced yard behind it. When you step out into that yard, you realize all you see is emotional junk. The whole backyard is filled with bad things that have happened in your life—physical or sexual abuse, emotional beatings, divorce, loss and disappointment.

Junk will always stink

In your efforts to work through these issues, you may have already spent years in this backyard. You've dug up every inch of that junk, looked it over and studied parts of it closely. Perhaps you've rearranged it, sorted it or tried to bury it deeper. But no matter what you do, you can't get rid of those bad things. They remain a part of your life and, unfortunately, they will always stink.

During the years of working on that yard, you may have picked up some insights or learned a lot about yourself. But at some point, you need to complete the learning and move on. When the time is right, make a clear decision to leave the junk in the backyard.

Plant flowers instead

Close the back door tightly, turn around and walk out the front door. Take a deep breath, enjoy the sunshine, then start planting flowers. In your front yard, cultivate a wide variety of beautiful things—kindness, patience, joy, excitement and talent.

Rather than holding on to your anger or grief or bitterness, decide on areas where you need to do additional work. Then leave the rest dormant in the backyard and focus on moving forward in your life.

Of course, the backyard will always stay hidden behind the house. But digging around in junk every day doesn't make you better. If you need to, once in a while go look into the yard and say, "Yes, that's a lot of junk!" Then leave it there, close the door, and go back to your flowers.

TODAY

- Create a short list of junk items or events in your "backyard."

- Write the words, "That's all junk and I'm leaving it there."

- Create a list of flowers or beautiful things in your front yard.

ஒ DAY 89 ஒ
I'm so angry

In spite of your efforts to prevent mean people from adding to your stress, sometimes you just can't escape their assault. Once in a while, people and situations make you furious. So what do you do when anger builds to the point of explosion?

Most people are uncomfortable with anger and avoid it as much as possible. We fear anger because it has the ability to destroy us. And if we really let go in expressing it, we know anger can cause damage that's hard to repair.

But what are you supposed to do with anger? If you don't have an acceptable outlet for it, anger quickly shoves you toward using food to keep it quiet.

Anger happens!
When you are verbally assaulted or harmed by someone, you are entitled to feel angry. But are you fretting over predicaments and wasting a lot of energy on things you can't change? When someone cuts you off in traffic or treats you rudely in a grocery store, do you really have to carry that burden home and take it to bed with you later?

Certainly, taking deep breaths, counting to ten or taking a walk will help decrease the intensity of your anger. But you can also learn other ways to handle anger "on the spot" and prevent it from building and getting worse. While coping with it won't resolve the issue that caused the anger, at least you'll be able to manage your feelings without blowing up or looking for something to eat.

I'm angry and I'm also...

When you reach for food to appease anger, you might be fixing the wrong emotion.

Here's a great way to identify what's going on besides anger. On a piece of paper, write, "I'm angry and I'm also..." then make a list of other emotions you are feeling such as disappointed, hurt or frustrated.

If you lost your job, you might also feel hurt, sad or worried. When your relationship ends, you might feel furious, devastated and lonely. And when you gain weight, you might feel disgusted, hopeless, uneasy or confused.

By paying attention to other emotions besides anger, you'll get a more accurate picture of the situation and why it upsets you. That will also help you work on dealing with those feelings instead of just feeling angry.

TODAY

- Identify a recent or past time when you felt intense anger.

- Write, "I'm angry and I'm also..." then list other emotions you were feeling.

- Create a plan for dealing with the emotions that weren't actually anger.

✄ DAY 90 ✁

Bitterness and resentment

After 18 years of marriage, Shannon's husband left her. She was devastated. But within a few weeks, her sadness and anger shifted into raging bitterness. To cope with her fury, she began shoving her feelings down by eating more. Day after day, she consumed lots of pastries and other comforting foods until her weight climbed to over 300 pounds.

Because she couldn't let go of feeling abandoned and rejected, Shannon continued to suffer for years. Long after her ex-husband remarried and moved to another state, she still couldn't forgive him or stop hating him. Without a way to get back at him, she turned to food as an outlet for her disappointment and hurt.

When she came to me for help, she immediately blamed her husband for her weight gain. "Look at what he did to me!" she sobbed. I gently responded, "No, Shannon. Look at what you did to you."

Over many months, we unraveled her deep feelings of bitterness and resentment. She slowly realized how her anger kept damaging her own life but had no effect on him. Through her journal, her sessions with me and her church women's group, Shannon was able to let go of her bitter feelings and allow herself to heal. At that point, she also began to successfully lose weight.

Bitterness grows

When you ignore feelings of hurt or push them away, they tend to become deeper, eventually growing into bitterness and resentment. The longer you hold these feelings, the harder it becomes to heal a wound. After a while, hurt builds into a chasm of resentment you can't escape from.

But in reality, when you insist, "I'll never forgive that person," you sentence yourself to an emotional prison. You think you've gotten justice and punished the guilty one. But instead of getting even, you become the victim. The other person doesn't feel the intense hurt or pain you want them to. Instead, you sacrifice your own health and your weight loss for the sake of staying angry and bitter.

To recover from bitterness, you have to be willing to process, feel, cry, let go and then do it all over again. Remember that healing comes slowly and incrementally. Like the turtle creeping toward the finish line, eventually you'll look back and see the progress you've made.

TODAY

- Identify times when you've been hurt or let down by another person.

- Write about your feelings around this, including any bitterness or resentment.

- Identify steps that will help you move toward recovery and healing.

DAYS 81–90 COMPLETED!

You've come this far in your 100 days...

Don't stop now. If you're struggling to stick with it, push yourself to finish *one more day*. You'll immediately be another day closer to achieving your weight-loss goals.

Just do one more day!

❧ DAYS 91–100 ❧

CREATE MAINTENANCE

❧ DAY 91 ❧

It's up to me!

One of my favorite studies on weight-loss success was done years ago by psychologists Robert Colvin and Susan Olson. For this project, they interviewed hundreds of people who had successfully lost weight and kept it off.

The standards for the study were tight, but they identified a significant number of people who were successful. Their participants had lost between twenty to 275 pounds and had maintained their goal weight an average of six years.

After doing many weight-loss programs that never brought lasting results, the study participants reached a similar conclusion. Ultimately, their secret to success came down to one word—ownership. They all used a variation of the phrase, "I had to figure out what worked for me and then I had to do it."

Own your program

Strict diets or rigid programs may help you lose weight, but to achieve long-term success, you have to own your plan as well as your results. That means you have to learn what works for you and keep those things in place forever.

With ownership, you stop blaming others for your failures and, instead, figure out strategies for coping better in the future. You also eliminate "if only" excuses such as, "If only I had more time, more money, a new job or a supportive spouse, I'd be able to stay on my diet."

You make it happen

Think carefully about what works in your current program. For example, evaluate the best time and method for your exercise. Decide if you need structure by planning your meals ahead of time and writing it out each day. Identify foods or snacks that you need to keep readily available.

Now think about what doesn't work. Perhaps you don't want a plan with too much flexibility but you also don't do well with a rigid, rule-based system. Maybe you realize that eating out so many nights tends to pull you off your program.

Remember that ownership involves figuring out what works as well as what doesn't work. You also need to do the actions that are right for you, not for someone else. Once you master the concept of ownership, you'll be amazed at how it will improve your outcomes.

TODAY

- Create a list of what works for you with your eating and exercise plans.

- Now make a list of what doesn't work and how you can avoid doing those things.

- Consider how to own your plan and make it personal for your own needs.

❧ DAY 92 ❧
How not to maintain

Helen couldn't figure out maintenance. "I don't know what went wrong!" she said. "I worked so hard to lose weight but now, look at me! I've gained it all back plus a bunch more. I do great when I'm dieting, but I guess I've never learned how to maintain."

I suspected it wasn't lack of knowledge that caused Helen to regain weight. She knew it all—from reciting the calorie content of almost any food to monitoring her target heart rate and choosing the ideal number of reps on her weight machine.

Things that don't work

The problem wasn't that Helen didn't know how to maintain. It was that she also knew exactly how not to maintain. I asked Helen to make a list of all the activities and behaviors that she knows don't keep her weight off. Here's what she came up with:

- Let my exercise program go. Stop taking walks.
- Watch a lot of TV, especially in the evenings.
- Drink more alcohol to relax.
- Spend time with my eating and drinking friends.
- Skip all my self-care or nurturing activities.
- Convince myself I don't care about my weight.
- Talk to my mother every day. (This always makes me want to eat.)

As she reviewed her list, Helen realized that she'd been doing the exact opposite of all the things that would help

202

maintain. Then I asked Helen to flip all of the items into positive actions that would bring long-term success.

For example, instead of watching TV all evening, she could fill her time with other activities she enjoyed. She listed her weekly scrapbooking group, home decorating projects and reading historical novels, which are her favorite type of books.

With each of the other things on her list, Helen planned how she could flip the activity into something that was much healthier for her weight management. Suddenly she got it! Helen realized she really did know how to maintain.

Make your own list of things that cause you not to maintain or stay on your diet plan. Then flip the list by stating each item in a positive way. Read your new list every day, and remind yourself that you absolutely do know how to maintain your weight.

TODAY

- Make a list of behaviors and activities that might cause you to gain weight back.

- Flip each item by stating it in a positive way or one that would help you maintain.

- Put three things from your list into action today. Record the outcome.

❧ DAY 93 ❧
How to eat right

Cheryl had been on a great weight-loss plan and was doing well. But she worried that once she went off her diet, she'd be in trouble because she never learned how to eat right. I suggested that instead, she probably knew a lot about not eating right. Together we made a list of the things she knew were not good habits or patterns:

- Skip breakfast, eat a salad for lunch, and be way too hungry when I get home.
- Eat junk foods instead of healthy things.
- Buy chips and cookies instead of fruits and vegetables. Not stock the kitchen with foods that I know are healthy.

Next, we made a list of what Cheryl knew about eating right:

- A candy bar does not replace a piece of fruit.
- A steak is not a vegetable. It gives you lots of protein, but it doesn't replace the nutrients and variety of fruits and vegetables.
- A large pizza is not a reasonable portion amount for one person.

Cheryl laughed when I asked if she knew what a carrot or an apple looked like. "Of course," she said. "I just avoid eating them because chocolate tastes better and is more fun." I agreed wholeheartedly. But loving the taste of non-healthy foods isn't the same as saying you never learned how to eat right.

Healthy eating guidelines

Like Cheryl, I'm sure you do know how to eat right. But here are a couple of basic guidelines to keep in mind.

1. Limit fried foods, sweets and desserts, chips and other snack foods. Notice I didn't say never eat these foods, but be careful about the amounts and how often you eat them.

2. Eat fruits and vegetables daily. You know what they are, so don't pretend you've never heard of these foods.

3. Learn the best portion amounts for you and your weight-loss plan. At restaurants, use the "half off special" which means you eat half as much as you really want or half the amount you might normally eat.

You can certainly improve your eating patterns by reading good diet books, making new recipes or exploring different types of food. Just be sure to focus on what you do know about healthy eating and then build it into your daily life.

TODAY

- Create your own list of ways to eat right.

- Check your supplies of fruits, vegetables and healthy meal options.

- Put your "eating right" plan in place today. Write down what you did.

✤ DAY 94 ✤
Don't say these things

A t lunch today, I cheated on my diet and then I blew it the rest of the day."

"I'd been so good all morning but this afternoon, I was really bad."

"Sometimes, I just can't resist temptation. And when I have a bad day, I can't stay on my diet."

Sound familiar? Unfortunately, these dieting phrases don't actually change your behavior. Instead, they reinforce your sense of failure and often make things worse. It's time to eliminate these five phrases and use healthier ones instead.

1. I cheated on my diet

The truth is, you can't cheat with food! The word *cheat* refers to something illegal or immoral, and food is neither of these. Instead, use the words *choose* or *choice* to describe your behaviors. You made a choice to eat that cookie, even if you wish you hadn't. Tomorrow, choose not to eat one.

2. Blew it

Saying "I blew it" gives you an open invitation to eat all evening and start your diet over tomorrow. If you slip up on your eating plan, call it a pause. This soft, non-judgmental word labels a mistake as a minor event instead of a crisis. After your pause, you simply return to your diet and get back on track.

3. I was good

Don't apply behavioral codes to what you do with food. You aren't good when you eat an apple, then bad because you chase it with a few cookies. And whether or not you stay on your diet has nothing to do with your being a good or a bad person.

4. I was bad

So where did you learn that a carrot was good and a brownie was bad? In most cases, you simply draw from a page showing allowed or not allowed foods, then chastise yourself for eating from the wrong list. Instead of calling yourself good or bad, refer to your food choices.

5. I can't...

"I can't resist Mom's apple pie or stay on a diet over the weekend." Every time you tell yourself you can't do something, you cement it as truth. Instead of saying, "I can't," switch to, "I'll find a way." By saying, "I'll find a way to stay on my diet," you strengthen your resolve to make it happen.

TODAY

- Which of the phrases in this lesson are you most likely to say? Write them down.

- Draw a line through those phrases to indicate you won't say them anymore.

- For each one, create a positive phrase that's the opposite of the old one.

❧ DAY 95 ❧
No birthday cake

My birthday is January 13th. And it's always the best day of my life. For many years, I would wake up feeling sluggish and depressed the day after my birthday. Finally, I realized that my usual birthday routine included doing things that would possibly shorten my life instead of lengthen it. So I made a decision to change the way I celebrate.

Each year, I proclaim my birthday as a day of ultimate self-care. This means that I intentionally do things that enhance my health and well-being. I make sure that I exercise, even if it's just a twenty-minute walk. I pay extra attention to eating in healthy ways and remind myself about having a piece of fruit and drinking plenty of water.

Sometimes, I treat myself to a massage or a manicure. I also make time for an afternoon cup of tea along with reading or other nurturing activities. And finally, I make sure that I play a few songs on my piano—an activity that I truly love.

No birthday cake!

Here's the most important thing. I rarely eat cake or dessert on my birthday anymore. This has become a great way to remember my ultimate goal, which is taking good care of myself.

The best part of celebrating my birthday this way is that at the end of the day, instead of feeling depressed about being another year older, I usually feel great. And the next year when my birthday comes around again, I'll follow the same plan, including labeling that day as the best day of my life.

When your next birthday comes, make it part of your healthy plan for the year and celebrate by doing some amazing self-care. Who knows? It might even make you feel younger instead of a year older!

Who will you eat cake for?

When celebrating other people's birthdays, do you feel obligated to eat birthday cake or dessert? If so, decide which people you will eat cake for. You might eliminate anyone who isn't a relative or all children under the age of six. You certainly don't have to compromise your eating goals just because a co-worker becomes a year older. You may discover you don't miss eating cake for people you aren't that close to.

TODAY

- Locate your next birthday on a calendar and write, "Ultimate self-care day."

- Create a list of things you will do that day for nurturing and self-care.

- Decide which people in your life you will eat cake for. If someone is not on your list, skip the birthday cake.

∽ DAY 96 ∾
Pull yourself back up

Most of us go through times when we feel down. You aren't really depressed but you just feel pulled down by things in your life. This vague sensation makes you yearn for foods that will help you feel nurtured and energized.

Instead of reaching for ice cream or chocolate, use this five-step plan to pull yourself back up. These steps take very little time but produce amazing results. The power comes from the completion of all five steps, so don't skip any of them. And while you don't have to do them in the order they are listed, following the sequence will reset your brain patterns and give you better results.

Step 1. Do tasks

Choose mundane tasks that don't require much thought or making decisions. Clear off your desk, sort the pile of old mail and magazines, clean out the coat closet or the junk drawer.

Step 2. Make music

Pull out some of your favorite inspiring or entertaining music. Crank it up loud and let the sound flow into your body. If you have the skills, play the piano or guitar. Sing along with the radio. Soak up the music and allow it to heal your spirit.

Step 3. Get active

Walk, run, ride a bike or do part of an aerobics or yoga routine. Dance in your living room or jump rope on the lawn. Find a way to move your body for at least ten minutes.

Step 4. Read a book

Choose a novel, a biography or a book of poetry. Perhaps read the Bible or a related inspirational book. Stay away from self-help books. The purpose here is to give your brain input, not make it do any work.

Step 5. Reflect

Sit in a quiet place and intentionally fill your mind with positive images or thoughts. Meditate, pray or do a visualization exercise. Invite your worries to leave and peacefulness to fill its place.

Any time clouds settle over you and make you long for the soothing comfort of pies and cookies, pull out this list and repeat the five steps. Keep the list handy and if you need it, do the steps daily for a while.

TODAY

- Write out your plan for the five steps. Include your own resources such as books or music.

- Even if you aren't feeling down, do the five steps at some point today.

- Record your response to this exercise, including how you felt afterward.

✎ DAY 97 ✎
Music therapy

It happens to all of us. No matter how hard you try, you can't stay on your diet longer than a few hours. You keep laying out your exercise clothes, but something always comes up and you never reach the gym or head out the door for your walk.

What if there is a secret ingredient that could boost you back into action? The answer is probably right in front of you. Whether you need to renew your spirit or calm a storm, listening to music provides a wonderful, non-food way to cope with feelings or brighten your mood.

The mood fix

Music can actually alter your body's physical and emotional state. In response to the beat of a song, your body shifts your heart rate, blood pressure and breathing to mimic the rhythm of the music. In fact, you can intentionally change your mood simply by choosing songs with the right beat.

For example, if you feel tired, depressed or lonely, skip the romantic ballads or slow country songs. Instead, listen to bright, forceful pieces with a fast tempo such as oldies or band marches.

For times when you need to calm down or soothe away anger, select music with a gentle rhythmic sound. Look for instrumental recordings, classical works or any quiet, relaxing music. Breathe slowly and deeply as you listen, allowing the music to lull you into a calmer state of mind.

The exercise link

If you've ever participated in aerobic exercise classes, you've seen what music can do. Music pumps you up, fuels your energy and keeps you going when you're tired or ready to quit. Not only does music entertain you and prevent boredom, it may even help you work out harder.

Studies have shown that people who listen to music while exercising stay with their activity longer than those who don't listen to music. It seems that your favorite tunes may be the key to better, more effective workouts.

Instead of reaching for food after a bad day, give yourself a musical escape. Lie on the floor and listen to your favorite music through headphones or earbuds. Immerse yourself in the sound, noticing the way it vibrates and is absorbed into your body. After five or ten minutes of music, you'll feel amazingly healed and revived.

TODAY

- Create a list of your favorite music to have readily available for times you need it.

- For at least ten minutes today, listen to music and focus on the beat.

- Record how it affects your energy and your spirit.

✎ DAY 98 ❧
Instant self-esteem

"It was an awful week!" Shelly said. "It started going bad when I found out I didn't get the new position at work." She reached for a tissue and wiped her eyes, then continued, "I thought I'd done everything right, but somehow it wasn't enough. When my boss told me the news, my confidence hit rock bottom."

Shelly sighed. "That afternoon, I went home and started eating and I don't think I've stopped since! Last night, my boyfriend and I had a terrible fight, and I know it was because I was so down on myself. My weight is totally out of control, my self-esteem is shot, and I feel like a failure in everything!"

"I'm so sorry that happened," I responded. "It sounds like you were devastated by the job issue, and I certainly don't blame you a bit. But what surprises me is the way you let this destroy so many other areas in your life as well."

Rebuild quickly

Just like Shelly, no matter how much you've worked on building your self-esteem, even a simple comment can devastate your inner spirit and send you running toward the refrigerator.

By making a few simple changes in your self-talk and your internal beliefs, you can improve your self-esteem very quickly. Silly, but effective, here's a quick exercise that will instantly boost your self-esteem. Read these three phrases in rapid succession, out loud if possible:

"I have sparkling eyes, I have a warm smile, and I'm going to make it!"

Repeat the entire sequence of phrases several times. You will be amazed at how it improves your mood. When you say, "I have sparkling eyes" several times in a row, your brain picks up the message and actually makes your eyes sparkle. The same is true with saying "warm smile."

You can vary the last phrase to match situations such as conducting a meeting, going on a job interview or preparing for a date. Just substitute words such as "I'm going to be great" or "I'm going to do my absolute best."

Plan to do this exercise every day for a week and notice how it affects your outlook. You'll be amazed at how much this simple exercise will change your self-esteem and improve your eating patterns.

TODAY

- Write the words from the "sparkling eyes" sentence on a card or in your journal.

- Read the phrases three times in a row, out loud if possible.

- Look for a time each day when you can recite the sentence. Record how this affects you.

✎ DAY 99 ✎
Do the work

In my coaching practice, I've watched many clients be successful long-term with managing their weight. Sadly, others struggle a lot and eventually gain it all back. The difference between these two groups usually comes down to one critical choice: Successful clients are willing to do the work.

For most of you, doing the work involves overcoming the barriers and excuses that keep you from your goals. You also have to learn how to manage life without using food as a solution. And you have to do these things for the rest of your life.

How to do the work

Here's how some of my clients described doing the work.

Carolyn: "I carried old beliefs that I'm not good enough or that things are my fault and I've done something wrong. I had to let go of those messages before I could stop turning to food for solace and comfort."

Ruth: "Whenever I left the nursing home after visiting my ill mother, I would stop at a fast-food restaurant. I had to work through my grief about her illness and, eventually, her death instead of eating it away."

Molly: "I had to learn to feel again. To the world, I looked fine, but inside I was living like a robot. I used Linda's exercise 'I feel, because of…' every day, and it helped me find back my emotions instead of shoving them down with food."

Sheila: "I had to stop taking the easy path. My daily routine included a couple glasses of wine every night, ice cream at bedtime and skipping exercise. I realized I was 'coping' every day instead of being willing to make my life better."

Alice: "I blamed other people and my life situation for not being able to lose weight. After going through some major health issues, I decided it was up to me to figure out how to take care of myself. I wish I had done it sooner."

I won't tell you that it's easy to do the work because it's not! Everyone struggles with this at times, including me. But when you keep pushing yourself to do the work, you'll be amazed at what you can accomplish with your weight-loss goals.

TODAY

- Identify the barriers and excuses that get in the way of your success. Make a decision that you will do the work to overcome them.

- Determine what's needed for doing the work in these areas. Write a plan for this.

- Do at least one thing today that demonstrates that you are doing the work.

❧ DAY 100 ❧
Weight-loss joy

You've reached a fork in the weight-loss road. If you follow one path, you'll continue to use the tools from this book. You'll also keep studying and learning about ways to reach and maintain your goals. On this road, you'll keep doing those things every day for the rest of your life. And, almost guaranteed, you'll become a long-term success story.

However, you can also choose to take a path that follows a gentle downhill slope. On this path, you'll probably return to many of your old habits and behaviors, and the odds are good that you'll start to regain the weight you worked so hard to lose.

Eventually, you'll be back at the same place as before, and desperately wishing you could lose some weight. So take a deep breath, picture your future and decide which path you will follow.

Creating weight-loss joy

One of the lessons from *100 Days of Weight Loss* describes the difference between being interested and being committed to managing your weight. Being committed means you stick with it, no matter what. It also means you take responsibility for your own actions and you keep going in spite of setbacks and problems.

When you remain committed, you learn how to enjoy the good times and survive the challenges. No matter what happens in your life, you continue to stay strong and positive about your journey. This is weight-loss joy! It's how you feel when it works! And I promise—you can do it.

Maintaining a healthy weight long-term doesn't happen automatically. Instead, you create this every single day by your plans, your thoughts and your actions. Regardless of where you are in your journey, you can live in an attitude of weight-loss joy.

So today, focus your energy on living from the place of joy in your heart. Draw from your deep well of skills and motivation tools and use them to frame the outline for your life. Certainly you will go through tough times when illness, stress or loss might creep in and pull you off track. But you have the power to minimize the damage and stay on the road.

Remind yourself to stand tall, breathe deeply and rehearse your affirmations and self-talk. Say things such as, "I can do this, I am strong and committed, and I'm living in weight-loss joy." Then go through every day with a powerful image of long-term success!

TODAY

- Define what your weight-loss joy looks like.

- Choose one specific way you'll live that out today.

- Record your thoughts on concluding this book.

DAYS 91–100 COMPLETED!

Congratulations!

You've made it through all 100 MORE days.

Now it's time for you to become a long-term success!

You've finished the 100 MORE Days of Weight Loss Program! But don't stop now! Think about what you need to do next. Would it help to repeat the 100 MORE Days lessons to cement them more strongly into your life? Do you need to focus on your top ten skills for a while until they become routine in your days?

Make sure you integrate all of the things you've learned into a daily, lifetime plan that will help you maintain your weight. Then keep learning more and adding to your skills.

Always remember the words, "A decision about what to weigh is a decision about how to live." If you follow this principle and use your skills and tools every single day, long-term success is practically guaranteed!

✺ INDEX ✺

❧ ABOUT THE AUTHOR ❧

Linda Spangle, RN, MA, is a weight-management coach recognized nationally as a leading authority on emotional eating and other psychological issues of weight loss. She is the author of three award-winning books: *Life Is Hard, Food Is Easy*, *100 Days of Weight Loss* and *Friends with the Scale*.

A registered nurse with a master's degree in health education, Linda is a skilled teacher, counselor and writer. She is the owner of Weight Loss for Life, a healthy lifestyles coaching and training program.

In addition to being interviewed by hundreds of radio shows, newspapers and magazines, Linda has been a guest on numerous TV shows including Fox News and Lifetime TV. She has been quoted in nearly every major women's magazine, including *Shape, Redbook, Women's Day* and *O Magazine*.

Linda is available for speaking engagements, training seminars and one-on-one weight-loss coaching. For information on her books and coaching programs as well as contact information, visit:

www.WeightLossJoy.com

100 MORE Days of Weight Loss
is also available in the following formats:

ebook – www.amazon.com
audio – www.amazon.com

❧ FREE MATERIALS ❧

Be sure to sign up for the free
support materials for this book.

www.100MOREdays.com

- 100 More Days printable journal
- 7 keys to successful weight loss
- Printable signs for lesson reminders
- Dot calendar for visually tracking your progress
- Extensive word list to help identify emotions

A printed version of

100 MORE Days of Weight Loss
Day-by-Day Journal

is available on www.amazon.com

OTHER BOOKS BY LINDA SPANGLE

Available in bookstores, Amazon.com and
www.WeightLossJoy.com

Life Is Hard, Food Is Easy
The 5-Step Plan to Overcome Emotional Eating
This book will completely change the way you think about
food, giving you a powerful strategy for conquering emotional
eating and other barriers to your success.

100 Days of Weight Loss
The Secret to Being Successful on ANY Diet Plan
These simple, day-by-day lessons will keep you focused and
committed to your weight-loss program for a minimum of
100 days.

Friends with the Scale
How to Turn Your Scale into a Powerful Weight Loss Tool
Based on stories and examples along with scientific data, this
book shows you how to discover the weight-loss power that
lies within your scale when you simply make it your friend.

Shaker Jar Diet
How to Use a Meal Replacement Plan to Lose Weight Fast
This book provides education and support for ANY brand
of meal-replacement program including Medifast®, HMR®,
Optifast® and many others.

LINDA SPANGLE'S WEBSITES

www.WeightLossJoy.com

Find details about Linda's books and weight-loss coaching programs as well as her extensive Media Room and contact information.

www.DietCoachCafe.com

Linda's library of FREE training materials, audio programs and resources including the Weight Loss Mastery Program.

www.TheDietQuiz.com

Based on your weight-loss goals, age, body type and preferences, this quiz guides you to the diet that's right for you.